AF223575

Silva
SUPERSTARS'
WEIGHT LOSS SECRETS

FROM THE MIND OF

José Silva

Silva SUPERSTARS' WEIGHT LOSS SECRETS

José Silva and Ed Bernd Jr.

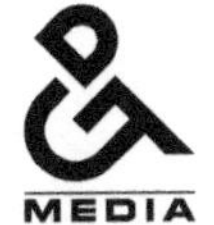

Published 2026 by Gildan Media LLC
aka G&D Media
www.GandDmedia.com

SILVA SUPERSTARS' WEIGHT LOSS SECRETS. Copyright © 2026 by Jose Silva and Silva Method UltraMind LLC. All rights reserved. The Silva Method is the registered trademark of Silva International Inc.

No part of this book may be used, reproduced or transmitted in any manner whatsoever, by any means (electronic, photocopying, recording, or otherwise), without the prior written permission of the author, except in the case of brief quotations embodied in critical articles and reviews. No liability is assumed with respect to the use of the information contained within. Although every precaution has been taken, the author and publisher assume no liability for errors or omissions. Neither is any liability assumed for damages resulting from the use of the information contained herein.

Front Cover design by David Rheinhardt of Pyrographx

Interior design by Meghan Day Healey of Story Horse, LLC.

Library of Congress Cataloging-in-Publication Data is available upon request

ISBN: 978-1-7225-0768-8

10 9 8 7 6 5 4 3 2 1

Contents

Chapter 1

Superstars' Weight Loss Secrets

Are you ready for a weight loss program that works . . . permanently? You've got one now, and all you need to do is relax and let the Silva Method guide you to guide your body—by natural means—to balance and adjust to a slim, sleek, fit, and healthy body the way nature intended. You will do this faster and more effectively if you avoid diet pills and other drugs, if you avoid crash diets and all the other forced weight loss methods.

Most weight loss programs don't work, at least not for very long. And there's a simple reason for that: They involve something from the outside, that tries to force you to do something you don't want to do.

You want to eat—that's a natural biological urge, for your survival. You want to taste something good, that brings you pleasure—that's a natural psychological urge, and is also part of your survival programming. You also want to feel good, to feel strong, healthy, and fit, and overeating can prevent that.

Most weight loss programs use force to try to overcome those natural urges to eat, to override that particular survival programming long enough for you to reduce your weight.

And you know all too well how that works: As soon as you reach your desired weight, the external weight loss program is no longer powerful enough to overcome those strong urges, that are generated by your survival programming; since you have reached the weight you wanted, the weight loss program is no longer able to force you to forgo the food and the pleasure—and your weight begins to climb right back up again.

The worst part is, the harder you fight to make these intrusive and abusive weight loss programs work, the less chance you have of success. The stronger the force, the more powerful the resistance. The more you use your "willpower" to avoid the food you desire, the more your "imagination" draws you right to it. And in any contest between the willpower and the imagination, the imagination always wins.

There is always a price to pay when you try to force yourself to do something against your natural urges:

Many people use drugs and upset their body chemistry, often with devastating—and sometimes even fatal—results.

Many people go on severe diets, often depriving themselves of nutrients they need as well as the eating pleasure they desire, and they become irritable and their family life suffers as they make life miserable for themselves and everybody else, because they are not healthy and fit.

There are substances that will block you up inside. Forced vomiting and powerful laxatives are sometimes used.

Some people even resort to surgery, using this violent and traumatic means of interfering with the body's natural processes and ripping out part of their body in their quest for their ideal weight and size.

And usually, it doesn't work—at least not in the long run.

Mind and Body Working Together to Get What You Want

Is there any good news in all this? Is there a method of weight loss that you can use to reach your ideal weight and size and then maintain that ideal weight and size?

Yes, there certainly is. And the best news is, you use only natural means; you do not have to force yourself; you do not have to do anything that you don't want to do. You work with your survival programming. And you work from the inside out. Like an artist, you create within yourself exactly the kind of body you desire, and you use completely natural methods in every phase of the process to make your dream a reality.

That's what the Silva Star Athlete, Superstars' Weight Loss Program is all about. This program was originally designed for the demanding needs of athletes, but it will work equally as well for anyone who applies it. We will guide you step by step through the entire program to ensure your success.

Countless people before you have succeeded in using the Silva techniques to reduce their weight and gain a body that people praise and admire, the body they've always wanted, and you will too, when you apply the simple techniques you will learn in this book.

The Silva Method got its start way back in 1944 when José Silva began researching, looking for ways to help his own children become as successful in life as he had become. Since 1966, when public seminars were first offered, millions of people worldwide, in 14 languages, have benefited from the Silva Method, just as you are about to benefit in your quest for your perfect body.

Imagination Is More Powerful Than Willpower

To help you understand how this is possible, let's take a look at how you, as a human being, function.

You have a body. You have a brain. You have a mind.

The brain is much like a computer that is programmed by the mind, or by what we will refer to as human intelligence.

The body is the vehicle that supplies the brain with fuel, with a means to get from one place to another, and with information it can use to solve problems and make decisions.

The mind is what makes us human, what permits us to change our environment and to create for ourselves all of the many things that we enjoy so much. Animals simply react to biological programming, programming that they are born with. Unless a human trains an animal, the animal will simply follow its natural urges.

When your body, brain, and mind are all functioning in harmony, then all is well and life is a genuine pleasure.

An animal cannot change its biological programming. But you can. With your mind, you can reprogram your biological computer—your brain—and by doing so, you can modify your biological urges.

You see, imagination—which is a function of your mind—is a double-edged tool:

When you use your imagination to imagine how much you will enjoy eating that gigantic chocolate sundae, with the cold ice cream and the hot chocolate fudge steaming away on top, and the crunchy nuts and the fluffy white whipped cream over everything—when you imagine all of this—then you want to go get it and eat it and enjoy the sweet taste in your mouth, and feel it sliding down your throat to give you that satisfied sensation of fullness and the knowledge that all is right with the world.

No amount of willpower can counteract that kind of an image. You have to fight fire with fire, as they say, and put your imagination to work to help you reach your goal.

The best part is, once you begin to learn how to control and direct your imagination, you can use it in all areas of your life to create results that seem like miracles.

All right, now that you've heard the bad news, and we've finished our discussion of why so many weight loss programs don't work, let's get started on the program that is going to get you the body you want.

First Step: Increase Your Motivation

Have you ever paused to list all of the reasons you have for wanting to reduce your weight? Most people have never actually done that.

Oh, you may realize you will be happier and will feel better if you lose weight. You probably have thought about the fact that you will be more popular.

But thoughts like that don't create the powerful, driving kinds of images and emotions that the thoughts of food create—like the mental picture we created a few minutes ago of the chocolate sundae. In order to use your imagination to help you reach your goal—your ideal weight and size—you have to create images that are just as powerful—and even more powerful than the images of food.

So let's begin with a list of reasons you have for wanting to reduce your weight.

First, get an exact image of what you want to look like.

Was there a time when you looked the way you want to look now? If so, recall how you looked then.

If you have a good picture of yourself, then get a copy of it and use it as a reminder. If not, then get a picture of somebody with the kind of body you desire and use it to create the image of yourself the way you want to look.

Since you are using a natural means of getting into the shape you want to be in, there are a couple of things you must keep in mind:

First, you must recognize that not everybody will look the same. You must consider your body type when you are setting your goals for your physical appearance.

Read the information in Chapter 9 to determine your body type. The best way to have a very attractive physique that will appeal to others is to work naturally with your own potential to bring out your best points.

A light-boned person can emphasize the slender fashion model physique, the sophisticated person moving in the best circles.

A heavy-boned person can develop a fuller, more sensuous physique that makes them extremely desirable partners.

The medium-boned person will find it easy to develop a dynamic athletic physique that communicates vibrant life.

You can't have all three. But you can easily have the one that your body is best suited for. And you can probably combine aspects of one of the other types of physique.

Awaken the Beauty That's Sleeping Within You

Some people are beautiful. Others are cute. Some are regal-looking. There is a look that invites you to come and have fun.

And there is a look that says the person is a winner, is in control, is a person you will be safe with. That kind of look, of course, is the most attractive of all, and it is a look you can develop whether you are beautiful or cute or handsome or rugged or whatever.

Remember the story of the ugly duckling? Discover the beautiful swan within you—or whatever beauty lies within you. Discover it, nurture it, enhance it, awaken the beauty that is sleeping within and use it to make your life the beautiful gift it was meant to be.

And let's exaggerate that image occasionally. After all, we tend to exaggerate our desire for food—we tend to exaggerate our problems—so let's exaggerate our goals, too, from time to time. Keep in mind, of course, the type of body you're looking for.

The second thing to remember is that if you have a long way to go, a long journey to take, take it one step at a time.

Can you imagine yourself at your ideal weight and size? Many people can't. One woman was programming to lose 50 pounds. When I asked her if she could honestly imagine herself 50 pounds lighter, she thought for a moment and then said, "No."

"Can you imagine yourself five pounds lighter?" I asked her.

She said she could do this, so she programmed to reduce her weight just five pounds. After that, she programmed to reduce another five pounds. With those successes behind her, she could believe that she could reduce 10 pounds, so that's what she programmed for next.

Eventually she reached her goal, one step at a time.

Can you believe you can reduce just one pound in the next week? And again the next week? And the next? If so, you can reduce 50 pounds in less than a year. And since you are doing it naturally, you will maintain that weight and size from now on, without fighting, without discomfort, without spending money for pills.

So for right now, get a specific dream in mind, the dream of that perfect body you desire, a practical dream based on the best possible use of your natural body type. When we begin the actual programming, we'll set our specific goals step by step until we are able to program believably for that dream and make it come true.

Let's pause for a moment before we continue, so that you can get two things: a picture of what you want to look like, one of yourself the way you want to look if you have one, or a picture of someone else you can use to remind you of your goal. Also, get paper and pen or pencil so you can write down some reasons for undertaking this Superstars' Weight Loss Program.

Put the book down now and get the picture, paper, and pencil or pen. When you are ready, pick up the book again and we'll start putting some real power into your desire to reduce your weight by using a technique that motivates the superstars.

How You Benefit from Reaching this Goal

It is important that you write out a list of reasons why you want to reach your goal. This is what puts the real power into your desire to succeed, and it will keep you going when you are tempted to quit.

The more reasons you have for reaching your goal, the greater will be your desire to succeed. That's one of the things that helps superstars achieve such outstanding results: They have such great desire to avoid failure, and to succeed.

There are social reasons to look your best. We have come through thousands of years of survival of the fittest, so it is only natural that we have some strong inborn programming to seek out a person who looks healthy and fit.

How will it help you to look healthy and fit, to look very desirable? Who will be interested? Why is this important to you?

Pause to write this down so you can use it later when you need to motivate yourself.

What about health? Would you like to live longer, and feel better every day of your life? Why would this be important to you? Would feeling healthier help you do more of the things you want to do? Would it help you in your interpersonal relationships—with family, on the job?

Remember to jot down these ideas as they come to you.

How else would you benefit: Save money on food? Be more in control of your own life, rather than letting food control you? Set a better example for your children?

Continue to practice this exercise from time to time. Whenever you happen to think of another reason to reduce your weight, write it down so you can use it later. You may think of another reason as you are going to sleep—write it down. You may think of a reason during a social activity, while eating breakfast, while working. Write down those reasons while you are thinking about them, and use them later to motivate yourself to reach your goals.

Take time now if you wish to write down some of your reasons for reducing your weight. When you are ready to continue with the book, you will learn how to use more of your brain and mind in a very special way, the way superstars do, to internalize these reasons so that you will begin to automatically desire these goals rather than desiring unnecessary food.

Chapter 2

How to Expand Your Consciousness and Use More of Your Mind

To begin, you will learn to relax and center yourself.

We spoke earlier of using imagination to create a perfect image of what you desire. And you have already gotten an actual picture to help you do that. But there is more to it.

You see, there is part of your brain that deals with the physical world, including food and hunger, and another part of the brain that deals with the mental world, including visualization and imagination.

Specifically, the left hemisphere of your brain stores memories of the physical world: what you see, what you hear, what you smell, taste, and feel. The right brain hemisphere is involved with visualization and imagination.

Your left brain hemisphere explains what you experience. It uses such things as language and numbers to represent the physical world.

Since your right brain hemisphere uses various kinds of images—form, shape, sound, movement—to experience the world, it experiences the world more directly.

To be successful, you need to use both. But most people, approximately 90 percent of humanity, use only the left brain hemisphere to think with.

You cannot tell by any "feeling" in your brain which side of the brain you are using. But you can learn to tell the difference. That's what you will be doing when you practice the Silva techniques.

How valuable is it to use both brain hemispheres to think with instead of just one? Well, suppose you thought you could only use one leg at a time. How much would that slow you down? How much would it interfere with your ability to get up and go to your car? Can a person with two legs run twice as fast as a person with one leg? Dance twice as well? A person with two legs can function much more than twice as good as a person with one leg. Of course, there are crutches and braces, but these are a poor substitute, just as starvation diets and strong drugs are a poor substitute for using your own natural abilities to reach your goals.

When you learn to use both sides of your brain to think with, this will do far more than double your ability to reach your goals.

Begin by Relaxing

How do you learn to use both sides of your brain to think with? First you relax your body, brain, and mind—without going to sleep. Then, when you are on the edge of sleep, you mentally repeat some beneficial statements and visualization and imagination exercises so you can learn to function in the subconscious consciously.

The relaxation exercise will guide you to enter the alpha brain wave level, where the gentle electrical pulsing of your brain is slowed to a level that corresponds to that of light sleep. But you won't go to sleep because you will be using your visualization and imagination.

When you are wide awake and physically active, the electrical energy of your brain probably vibrates about 20 times per second. That rate is known as beta brain wave frequency. In deepest sleep, it pulses less than once a second, the delta frequency. In light sleep, it is in the alpha range, about 10 vibrations per second.

The Silva Centering Exercise guides you to enter the alpha level without going to sleep, and then while at that level, you will begin to transfer memories from your left brain hemisphere to your right brain hemisphere so that you can change them, alter them, and create a blueprint, in a place in your brain where it will guide your body and your mind toward your goal.

Change from the Inside Out

Why do all this? You must first be at the alpha level to be able to use both your left and your right brain hemispheres to think with. Then you must transfer information from the left hemisphere to your right brain hemisphere so that it has something to begin to work with. It is like learning to use two brains instead of one.

Once you do that, and you are using the right brain hemisphere, you can use your mental senses, your visualization and imagination, to influence your body and to help control your appetite and your weight.

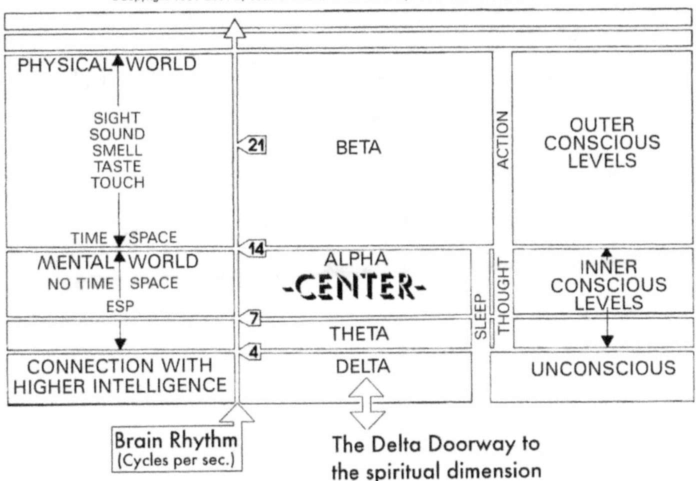

You can also learn other techniques, including ESP, to help you in all areas of your life: to improve your health, to improve your memory and your ability to pass tests, to improve your ability to earn money and have even more of the things you desire in life, to improve your relationships and your ability to find long-lasting love and happiness.

You can learn techniques to help you overcome specific problems like tension and migraine headaches. You can learn to control dreams and to use them to get information to solve problems. You can learn to improve your creativity and intuition, and much more.

If you'd like information on other Silva programs, please see the Resources in the Appendix at the end of the book.

For now, make yourself comfortable and we'll begin to learn to relax and enter the alpha level so you can use your right brain hemisphere to create the blueprints of that perfect body you desire.

Chapter 3

What Is the Alpha Level

Your brain is like a computer. It operates on a small amount of electricity. It can process information and experience and save them to use later.

The electricity of the brain vibrates—beats—at various rates, sometimes fast, sometimes slow. Scientists have grouped the vibrations and named them, based on how many vibrations (cycles) per second:

- 14 to 21 cycles per second = Beta
- 7 to 14 cycles per second = Alpha
- 4 to 7 cycles per second = Theta
- .5 to 4 cycles per second = Delta

As you can see, the halfway point—the center of the brain frequency spectrum—is in the center of the alpha range.

Alpha is usually just below the "outer conscious" level, in the area of light sleep, where we dream, but not the lower frequencies associated with deep sleep.

The beta brainwave level is associated with physical activity when we need to use our eyesight, so your brain wants to be at beta whenever you are using your physical eyesight or attempting to use your physical eyesight. That is why we advise you to keep your eyes closed when you are learning to function dynamically at the alpha level.

How to Find the Alpha Level

Finding the alpha level is easy. We have two ways to learn:

1. With the Silva Centering Exercise you move in the direction of sleep but maintain just enough mental activity to keep you from actually going to sleep.
2. With the second method you learn to re-enter the center of the alpha level after you first wake up.

The fastest way is to have someone read the Centering Exercise to you. You can also use a recording, either one you make yourself or one that somebody else made for you. You can find one at the SilvaNow.com website or by searching YouTube.com for Centering Exercise Ed Bernd Jr.

If you want to make your own recording, you can use the script in the next chapter.

The alternative way is simple to use but takes longer, 40 days. You can go to the Appendix of this book and follow the instructions.

If you want to proceed with the Centering Exercise then first read the next chapter.

Or you can use the alternative, the 40-day countdown system in the Appendix.

Chapter 4

Enter the Alpha Level with the Silva Centering Exercise

Please note: These mental exercises require that you close your eyes and relax physically and mentally; they must not be used while driving a car or performing other activities that require the use of eyesight.

To help ensure that you remain at the inner conscious level, we will practice these exercises with eyes closed.

When you are instructed to visualize and imagine tranquil and passive scenes, that means to use your memory to recall something you have seen before, or use your imagination and imagine what something looks like that you have never seen or imagined before.

When you are ready to begin, find a place where you can sit comfortably and won't be disturbed for about 30 minutes. Any position that is comfortable is a good position. During these exercises, you may change your position to make yourself more comfortable. You may do whatever is necessary to make yourself comfortable.

If you feel you must open your eyes, then do so and make yourself comfortable, but if you open your eyes, you must start over again after you have made yourself comfortable.

You must learn to concentrate and maintain your attention on what you desire to think about. If another thought intrudes, let it go and bring your attention back to what you desire.

Avoid making any effort in the mental dimension. You should not force yourself to relax. You need to learn to relax. Keep in mind that trying creates tension, and in the world of the mind, that makes matters worse. In the world of the mind you need to attract what you desire. Learn to relax, and concentrate on what you desire.

Chapter 5

Get the Body You Want with Your Subconscious Power

Once you learn to use your mind to relax your body, then it will be easy to learn to use your mind to reshape your body and to get the body you want.

It will also be easier to use your mind to help you recover from injuries and to overcome and avoid illnesses.

Then learn to relax your mind by visualizing—recalling—tranquil and passive scenes, and by projecting yourself mentally to your ideal place of relaxation, and then it will be easy to learn to project your mind to any point or place on the planet (and beyond) to detect information you can use to help you correct problems and achieve your goals.

Has your subconscious been kicking you around, making it hard for you to do what you know you should be doing to lose weight?

It is time for you to take charge and start using your subconscious power consciously instead of letting it control you.

What is this subconscious mind that psychologists speak of?

It is an area of the brain that is active during light sleep. The electrical energy powering the brain slows down when you go to sleep; it doesn't pulse as rapidly.

It also becomes more energetic and provides more power for mental activity because you are no longer using energy for physical activity.

Consciousness Expansion Simplified

"Most people have only learned two states of consciousness," José Silva said, "awake and asleep."

Now it is time to learn a third state of consciousness, what psychologists have named the "subconscious." The subconscious is just below the conscious level, and is associated with light sleep.

Memories and ideas that are stored in the "subconscious" part of the brain continue to influence you even though you are not consciously aware of them.

Would you like to go into this area and "reprogram" the old ideas that are not serving you well? That is what we will begin doing during the Silva Centering Exercise. Then we will give you more tools to work with in the next two mental training exercises.

First we need access to the so-called subconscious mind. One thing to remember is to avoid using your physical eyesight. Visualizing is remembering—remembering what something looks like. You don't need your physical eyesight for that.

We need our physical eyesight when we are interacting with the physical world, to help us become aware of danger so we can avoid it, and to see opportunities so we can take advantage of them. That is when we also need the beta part of our brain to be active.

So use your eyesight at the beta brainwave frequencies and your mind at the slower alpha frequencies.

After you have learned to use your mind at the alpha level with your eyes closed, then you can learn to function at alpha with eyes open when necessary. That is beyond the scope of this weight loss workshop, so we will save that for later.

Learning to use your subconscious consciously is also the key to unlocking your psychic ability.

We explain exactly how to do it in *José Silva's Everyday ESP Master Course* so you can learn to detect hidden information, influence people remotely, make better decisions, be more times right than wrong, and live the kind of productive, successful, and meaningful life you desire.

How to Find the Alpha Level

Q: What is the most effective Silva UltraMind exercise for beginners to access the alpha state?

A: José Silva said the most valuable thing he accomplished in his 22 years of scientific research, at a cost of half a million dollars (that's probably $2 million today when you adjust for inflation), was how to use the subconscious consciously. Most people, he said, have only two states of consciousness: conscious and unconscious (including sleep).

So the "secret" is to go to the same level—brain frequency-wise—as light sleep . . . but stay awake.

Choose the Method That Suits You Best

José Silva offered two ways to find the alpha (inner conscious) level:

1. Practice the Silva Centering Exercise. Do the things you do when you go to sleep, and condition yourself with "trigger mechanisms" so that in the future you can reach the alpha level instantly by using the trigger mechanisms.

What do you do when you are ready to go to sleep? You make yourself comfortable, close your eyes, relax physically and mentally . . . and fall asleep. In the Silva Centering Exercise you just follow those instructions. But add one more step: When you relax physically, associate that with the number 3. When you relax mentally, associate that with the number 2. Once you have relaxed physically and mentally and have that pleasant feeling when you wake up in the morning on your day off, you are at the alpha level—not quite awake, but not quite asleep. Associate that with number 1.

That process is known as classical conditioning (developed by a Russian scientist named Pavlov).

But won't you fall asleep? Not when you are repeating the beneficial statement; not when you are using visualization and imagination to recall tranquil and passive scenes; not when you are solving problems and creating solutions mentally. Just use your mind to recall what things look like (visualization and imagination) and not your physical eyes. Eyesight is for taking action in the beta world. Eyesight acts like a switch: When you attempt to focus your eyes to see something, your brain immediately goes to the faster beta brainwave frequencies. You can learn later how to function at alpha with your eyes open when necessary, but first learn to use alpha with your eyes closed.

2. The second way you can learn to function at alpha is to practice countdown-deepening exercises every morning when you first wake up for 40 mornings. You are just coming out of alpha when you wake up, so it will be easy to go back to alpha. The countdowns, along with the fact that your body has already had enough sleep, will help to ensure that you don't fall asleep again. Just keep visualizing the numbers as you count downward toward 1. That method is described in detail in several of the Silva books.

It isn't magic; it is science. You can easily learn to develop a third state of consciousness: Awake (conscious), Inner Conscious Level, Unconscious (asleep).

Some people tell you to turn your eyes upward when you meditate. Ignore them. You don't turn your eyes upward when you go to sleep at night do you? You don't do it when you are learning to enter the alpha level without going to sleep either.

Later, after you have learned to find the alpha level, there are situations where you can increase alpha production by turning your eyes slightly upward while using your visualization and imagination to correct problems.

Keep it simple and you will succeed. You can learn more with the Free Introductory Lessons at the SilvaNow.com website, our YouTube channel at youtube.com/@silvamindvideo and the Silva Centering Exercise in the next chapter.

Chapter 6

The Silva Centering Exercise

In order to expand your consciousness so that you can use the subconscious with conscious awareness, you need to do two things:

- Lower your brain frequency from its fully awake 20 cycles per second vibration rate to 10 cycles per second alpha frequency range.
- Then stay in alpha and do not go to the lower theta and delta frequencies associated with deep sleep.

José Silva found a simple way to do that. It involves a combination of classical conditioning along with something he learned from hypnosis.

Since your brain is already accustomed to going to alpha under certain circumstances, he hypothesized he could expand on that ability.

Going to Alpha Naturally

When does the brain slow to alpha? When you go to sleep.

What do you do before you go to sleep? You find a comfortable position. You close your eyes. You relax physically and mentally.

When you do that, your brain frequency starts slowing down . . . and . . . you go to sleep.

What can stop you from going to sleep but allow you to remain at the alpha level?

The same thing that kept his hypnosis subjects from going to sleep:

Provide a small amount of mental activity that will let you remain at the alpha frequency, but not something interesting enough to bring you back to the higher beta frequencies.

We give you simple tasks like visualizing tranquil and passive scenes.

We ask you to mentally repeat beneficial statements, for instance.

But at the very beginning we don't ask you to solve any problems.

This small amount of mental activity will help you stay at alpha and avoid continuing to lower frequencies.

Once you have learned to follow our simple instructions and remain at alpha, then it is easy for you to learn to analyze information and develop solutions while remaining at alpha.

Using the Silva Centering Exercise

What we just described is the Silva Centering Exercise (previously known as the Long Relaxation Exercise).

It is a "conditioning cycle" and "conditions" you to be able to relax physically and mentally and enter the alpha level in a matter of seconds.

You need to do more than just listen:

You need to follow the instructions in the conditioning cycle. Do what the instructor guides you to do.

In the Silva Centering Exercise, we ask you to make yourself comfortable, close your eyes, and relax your body from head to toes. Then we associate this physical relaxation to the number 3.

Then we guide you to relax mentally and associate mental relaxation to the number 2.

As you continue to follow the simple instructions, your brain will be at the alpha frequency. We associate this with the number 1.

After you have practiced a few times, you will be able to enter the alpha level in a few seconds by mentally repeating and visualizing the numbers with the intention of entering alpha. You will simply:

- Take a deep breath and, while exhaling, mentally repeat and visualize the number 3 three times, and *relax* physically.
- Take another deep breath and, while exhaling, mentally repeat and visualize the number 2 three times, and *relax* mentally.
- Take another deep breath and, while exhaling, mentally repeat and visualize the number 1 three times, and take it for granted that you have entered the alpha level.

Stay positive. Take it for granted that you are at the correct level.

Some people report that being at the alpha level is similar to how they feel when they first wake up from a restful night's sleep.

The fastest way to learn is to have someone guide you through the Silva Centering Exercise. You can have somebody read it to you or record it for you, or listen to a CD or mp3 audio, or steam it online, or you can record it yourself. The script follows.

You can start with the Free Introductory Lessons at the SilvaNow.com website. You can also find it on YouTube by searching for: Silva Centering Exercise Ed Bernd Jr.

How to Read the Silva Centering Exercise

José Silva has this advice for reading the Centering Exercise to another person or to make a recording you can listen to and let it guide you through the process:

"When reading the Silva Centering Exercise, read in a relaxed, natural voice. Be close enough so that the listener can hear you comfortably. Read loud enough to be heard, and read as though you were reading to a seven-year-old child. Speak each word clearly and distinctly.

"Have the listener assume a comfortable position. A sitting position is preferred, but the most important thing is to make sure the listener is comfortable. If uncomfortable, the listener will not relax as much and will not get as much benefit from the exercise.

"Avoid distractions, such as loud outside noises. There should be enough light so you can read comfortably, but not extremely bright lights.

"If the person shows any signs of nervousness or appears to be uncomfortable, stop reading; tell them to relax and make themselves comfortable. When they are comfortable and ready, then continue.

"Take your time when you read; there is no need to rush."

A Quick Review:

- Sit in any position that is comfortable; let your body do what it needs to do to be comfortable. It is okay to lie down if you need to.
- If you need to readjust your position, do so; if you need to scratch, scratch.
- If you need to open your eyes, then open your eyes and make yourself comfortable. Then when you are ready, close your eyes and start again at the beginning of the exercise.
- Follow the instructions. Don't just sit passively; get involved, and let your body relax.
- To "visualize the number 3" means to recall what it looks like. Use your mind, not your physical eyesight.

- Do the same to "detect a fine vibration, a tingling sensation, a feeling of warmth." Recall a sensation like that. Do it with your mind.
- To "release and relax all tensions and ligament pressures" is like releasing your grip on something you have been holding tightly. You cannot force yourself to relax, so just let go and relax your muscles.

The Silva Centering Exercise Script

Note: Do not read the headings out loud. They are for your information.

Deepening (Physical Relaxation at Level 3)

We will start this exercise with the 3 to 1 method.

Find a comfortable position, close your eyes, take a deep breath, and, while exhaling, mentally repeat and visualize the number 3 three times. (pause)

To help you learn to relax physically at level 3, I am going to direct your attention to different parts of your body.

Concentrate your sense of awareness on your scalp, the skin that covers your head; you will detect a fine vibration, a tingling sensation, a feeling of warmth caused by circulation. (pause) Now release and completely relax all tensions and ligament pressures from this part of your head and place it in a deep state of relaxation that will grow deeper as we continue. (pause)

Concentrate your sense of awareness on your forehead, the skin that covers your forehead; you will detect a fine vibration, a tingling sensation, a feeling of warmth caused by circulation. (pause) Now release and completely relax all tensions and ligament pressures from this part of your head and place it in a deep state of relaxation that will grow deeper as we continue. (pause)

Concentrate your sense of awareness on your eyelids and the tissue surrounding your eyes; you will detect a fine vibration, a tingling sensation, a feeling of warmth caused by circulation. (pause) Now release and completely relax all tensions and ligament pressures from this part of your head and place it in a deep state of relaxation that will grow deeper as we continue. (pause)

Concentrate your sense of awareness on your face, the skin covering your cheeks; you will detect a fine vibration, a tingling sensation, a feeling of warmth caused by circulation. (pause) Now release and completely relax all tensions and ligament pressures from this part of your head and place it in a deep state of relaxation that will grow deeper as we continue. (pause)

Concentrate on the outer portion of your throat, the skin covering your throat area; you will detect a fine vibration, a tingling sensation, a feeling of warmth caused by circulation. (pause) Now release and completely relax all tensions and ligament pressures from this part of your body and place it in a deep state of relaxation that will grow deeper as we continue. (pause)

Concentrate within the throat area and relax all tensions and ligament pressures from this part of your body and place it in a deep state of relaxation, going deeper and deeper every time. (pause)

Concentrate on your shoulders; feel your clothing in contact with your body. (pause) Feel the skin and the vibration of the skin covering this part of your body. (pause) Relax all tensions and ligament pressures and place your shoulders in a deep state of relaxation, going deeper and deeper every time. (pause)

Concentrate on your chest; feel your clothing in contact with this part of your body. (pause) Feel the skin and the vibration of your skin covering your chest. (pause) Relax all tensions and ligament pressures and place your chest in a deep state of relaxation, going deeper and deeper every time. (pause)

Concentrate within the chest area; relax all organs; relax all glands; relax all tissues, including the cells themselves, and cause them to function in a rhythmic, healthy manner. (pause)

Concentrate on your abdomen; feel the clothing in contact with this part of your body. (pause) Feel the skin and the vibration of your skin covering your abdomen. (pause) Relax all tensions and ligament pressures and place your abdomen in a deep state of relaxation, going deeper and deeper every time. (pause)

Concentrate within the abdominal area; relax all organs; relax all glands; relax all tissues, including the cells themselves and cause them to function in a rhythmic, healthy manner. (pause)

Concentrate on your thighs; feel your clothing in contact with this part of your body. (pause) Feel the skin and the vibration of your skin covering your thighs. (pause) Relax all tensions and ligament pressures and place your thighs in a deep state of relaxation, going deeper and deeper every time. (pause)

Sense the vibrations at the bones within the thighs; by now these vibrations should be easily detectable. (pause)

Concentrate on your knees; feel the skin and the vibration of your skin covering the knees. (pause) Relax all tensions and ligament pressures and place your knees in a deep state of relaxation, going deeper and deeper every time. (pause)

Concentrate on your calves; feel the skin and the vibration of the skin covering your calves. (pause) Relax all tensions and ligament pressures and place these parts of your body in a deep state of relaxation, going deeper and deeper every time. (pause)

To enter a deeper, healthier level of mind, concentrate on your toes. (pause) Enter a deeper, healthier level of mind.

To enter a deeper, healthier level of mind, concentrate on the soles of your feet. (pause) Enter a deeper, healthier level of mind. (pause)

To enter a deeper, healthier level of mind, concentrate on the heels of your feet. (pause) Enter a deeper, healthier level of mind. (pause)

Now cause your feet to feel as though they do not belong to your body. (pause)

Feel your feet as though they do not belong to your body. (pause)

Your feet feel as though they do not belong to your body. (pause)

Your feet, ankles, calves, and knees feel as though they do not belong to your body. (pause)

Your feet, ankles, calves, knees, thighs, waist, shoulders, arms, and hands feel as though they do not belong to your body. (pause)

You are now at a deeper, healthier level of mind, deeper than before.

This is your physical relaxation level 3. Whenever you mentally repeat and visualize the number 3, your body will relax as completely as you are now, and more so every time you practice.

Deepening (Mental Relaxation at Level 2)

To enter the mental relaxation level 2, mentally repeat and visualize the number 2 several times, and you are at level 2, a deeper level than 3. (pause) Level 2 is for mental relaxation, where noises will not distract you. Instead, noises will help you to relax mentally more and more.

To help you learn to relax mentally at level 2, I am going to call your attention to different passive scenes. Visualizing any scene that makes you tranquil and passive will help you relax mentally.

Your being at the beach on a nice summer day may be a tranquil and passive scene for you. (pause)

A day out fishing may be a tranquil and passive scene for you. (pause)

A tranquil and passive scene for you may be a walk through the woods on a beautiful summer day, when the breeze is just right, where there are tall shade trees, beautiful flowers, a very blue sky, an occasional white cloud, birds singing in the distance, even squirrels playing on the tree limbs. Hear birds singing in the distance. (pause)

This is mental relaxation level 2, where noises will not distract you.

To enhance mental relaxation at level 2, practice visualizing tranquil and passive scenes.

TO ENTER YOUR CENTER

To enter level 1, mentally repeat and visualize the number 1 several times. (pause)

You are now at level 1, the basic level where you can function from your center.

DEEPENING EXERCISES

To enter deeper, healthier levels of mind, practice with the countdown-deepening exercises. To deepen, count downward from 25 to 1, or from 50 to 1, or from 100 to 1. When you reach the count of 1, you will have reached a deeper, healthier level of mind, deeper than before.

You will always have full control and complete dominion over your faculties and senses at all levels of the mind, including the outer conscious level.

When to Practice

The best time to practice the countdown-deepening exercises is in the morning when you wake up. Remain in bed for at least five minutes practicing the countdown-deepening exercises.

The second-best time to practice is at night, when you are ready to retire.

The third best time to practice is at noon after lunch.

Five minutes of practice is good; 10 minutes is very good; 15 minutes is excellent.

To practice once a day is good; two times a day is very good; and three times a day is excellent.

If you have a health problem, practice for 15 minutes, three times a day.

To Come out of Levels

To come out of any level of the mind, count to yourself mentally from 1 to 5 and tell yourself that at the count of 5 you will open your eyes, be wide awake, feeling fine and in perfect health, feeling better than before.

Then proceed to count slowly from 1 to 2, then to 3, and at the count of 3 mentally remind yourself that at the count of 5 you will open your eyes, be wide awake, feeling fine and in prefect health, feeling better than before.

Proceed to count slowly to 4, then to 5. At the count of 5 and with your eyes open, mentally tell yourself, "I am wide awake, feeling fine, and in perfect health, feeling better than before. And this is so."

Deepening (Routine Cycle)

To help you enter a deeper, healthier level of mind, I am going to count from 10 to 1. On each descending number, you will feel yourself going deeper and you will enter a deeper, healthier level of mind.

10—9, feel going deeper
8—7—6, deeper and deeper
5—4—3, deeper and deeper
2—1

You are now at a deeper, healthier level of mind, deeper than before.

You may enter a deeper, healthier level of mind by simply relaxing your eyelids. Relax your eyelids. (pause) Feel how relaxed they are. (pause) Allow this feeling of relaxation to flow slowly downward throughout your body, all the way down to your toes. (pause)

It is a wonderful feeling to be deeply relaxed, a very healthy state of being.

To help you enter a deeper, healthier level of mind, I am going to count from 1 to 3. At that moment, you will project yourself mentally to your ideal place of relaxation. I will then stop talking to you, and when you next hear my voice, one hour of time will have elapsed at this level of mind. My voice will not startle you; you will take a deep breath, relax, and go deeper.

1—(pause)—2—(pause)—3. Project yourself mentally to your ideal place of relaxation until you hear my voice again. Relax. (**Reader**: remain silent for about 30 seconds.)

Relax. (pause) Take a deep breath and, as you exhale, relax and go deeper. (pause)

Rapport

You will continue to listen to my voice; you will continue to follow the instructions at this level of the mind and any other level, including the outer conscious level. This is for your benefit; you desire it, and it is so.

Whenever you hear me mention the word "relax," or whenever you mentally or verbally mention the word "relax," all unnecessary movements and activities of your body, brain, and mind will cease immediately, and you will become completely passive and relaxed physically and mentally.

I may bring you out of this level or a deeper level than this by counting to you from 1 to 5. At the count of 5, your eyes will open; you will be wide awake, feeling fine and in perfect health.

I may bring you out of this level or a deeper level than this by touching your left shoulder three times. When you feel my hand touch your left shoulder for the third time, your eyes will open; you will be wide awake, feeling fine and in perfect health. And this is so.

Genius Statements

The difference between genius mentality and lay mentality is that geniuses use more of their minds and use them in a special manner.

You are now learning to use more of your mind and to use it in a special manner.

Beneficial Statements

The following are beneficial statements that you may occasionally repeat while at these levels of the mind. Repeat mentally after me. (**Instructor**: read slowly.)

My increasing mental faculties are for serving humanity better.

Every day, in every way, I am getting better, better, and better.

Positive thoughts bring me benefits and advantages I desire.

I will always maintain a perfectly healthy body and mind.

I have full control and complete dominion over my sensing faculties at this level of the mind and any other level, including the outer conscious level. And this is so.

Effective Sensory Projection Statements

Effective Sensory Projection statements for success:

I am now learning to attune my intelligence by developing my sensing faculties and to project them to any point or place on this planet so as to be aware of any actions taking place, if this is necessary and beneficial for humanity.

I am now learning to attune my intelligence by developing my sensing faculties and to project them to any point or place on any planet within the solar system, any solar system within the galaxy, and any galaxy within the universe so as to be aware of any actions taking place, if this is necessary and beneficial for humanity.

I am now learning to attune my intelligence by developing my sensing faculties and to project them to the different matter kingdoms: the inanimate matter kingdom, any of its levels and depths; the animate matter kingdom with reproductive intelligence, plant life, and animal life, any of its levels and depths; and the animate matter kingdom with reproductive intelligence and an awareness of existence, the human body and mind kingdom, any of its levels and depths.

I am now learning to detect abnormalities whenever such abnormalities exist within any kingdom, any level, and any depth, if this is necessary and beneficial for humanity.

I am now learning to apply corrective measures and to bring back to normalcy any abnormality found within any kingdom, any level, and any depth, if this is necessary and beneficial for humanity.

Negative thoughts and negative suggestions have no influence over me at any level of the mind.

Post Effects: Preview of Next Session

You have practiced entering deep, healthy levels of mind. In your next session, you will enter a deeper, healthier level of mind, faster and easier than this time.

Post Effects: Standard

Every time you function at these levels of the mind, you will receive beneficial effects physically and mentally.

You may use these levels of the mind to help yourself physically and mentally.

You may use these levels of the mind to help your loved ones, physically and mentally.

You may use these levels of the mind to help any human being who needs help, physically and mentally.

You will never use these levels of the mind to harm any human being; if this be your intention, you will not be able to function within these levels of the mind.

You will always use these levels of the mind in a constructive, creative manner for all that is good, honest, pure, clean, and positive. And this is so.

You will continue to strive to take part in constructive and creative activities to make this a better world to live in, so that when we move on, we shall have left behind a better world for those who follow. You will consider the whole of humanity, depending on their ages, as fathers or mothers, brothers or sisters, sons or daughters. You are a superior human being; you have greater understanding, compassion, and patience with others.

Bringout

In a moment, I am going to count from 1 to 5. At that moment, you will open your eyes, be wide awake, feeling fine and in perfect health, feeling better than before. You will have no ill effects whatsoever in your head, no headache; no ill effects whatsoever in your hearing, no buzzing in your ears; no ill effects whatsoever in your vision and eyesight; vision, eyesight, and hearing improve every time you function at these levels of mind.

1—2, coming out slowly now.

3, at the count of 5, you will open your eyes, be wide awake, feeling fine and in perfect health, feeling better than before, feeling the way you feel when you have slept the right amount of revitalizing, refreshing, relaxing, healthy sleep.

4—5, eyes open, wide awake, feeling fine and in perfect health, feeling better than before.

(**Reader**: Be sure to observe whether or not the person is wide awake. If in doubt, touch the person's left shoulder three times and while doing so say: "Wide awake, feeling fine and in perfect health. And this is so.")

It is recommended that everyone practice staying at their center for 15 minutes a day to normalize all abnormal conditions of the body and mind.

If you would like to share this experience with family members, friends, and associates, please see the Save the Planet Project in Appendix B.

Chapter 7

Superstars' Weight Loss Programming

What kind of body do you want to have?

You can have it by using the Silva techniques, and a little bit of common sense.

Now that you've had the opportunity to learn to enter the alpha brain wave level, and to practice relaxing your body, brain, and mind with the Silva Centering Exercise, you're ready to begin programming to reduce your weight and to create the body you desire.

You must use the Centering Exercise at least four times, before you begin to use the programming exercise in the next chapter. And you need to continue to practice the Centering Exercise once or twice a week. When you practice it, be sure that you get involved in it, and relax yourself physically and mentally every time. This is very important.

You've already learned how you can use your mind to guide your body, and you have actually used your mind to relax your body. It is now just a short step to use your mind to help you control your weight.

Before we go on to the programming exercise, let's talk a bit about habits, programming, and human nature, so you will better understand what we are doing and why.

What Are Habits?

Habits are patterns of behavior, repeated over and over until they become automatic—until it becomes easier to do it than not to.

The body is very good at adapting to whatever load is placed on it, to almost any conditions. So is the mind. That's how habits are born. And the good news is, that's how habits can be changed.

We adapt physically. And we adapt psychologically. Cigarette smoking and drinking both cause severe irritation to a body that has not adapted to these harsh substances. Yet once we persist and adapt, and make a habit of using these things, then the body becomes irritated when it does not get them.

Overeating is not good for the body, especially when we eat too much saturated fat, refined sugars, and refined flour products. This can clog us up, impede blood flow to muscles and brain, and slow our physical reactions and our mental processes. It can make us overweight and unattractive, and virtual social outcasts. It can keep us from better jobs, can ruin our chances for the relationships we desire, sabotage our self-image and self-esteem, make us ill, and even kill us.

Who needs it? Nobody.

So why do we do it?

Habits such as overeating, drinking, and smoking are fueled by our survival mechanism, until eventually they take on a life of their own. They can all be highly addictive, both psychologically and physiologically. I'll explain.

Life is filled with opportunities. Sometimes these opportunities come in the form of challenges. And it is human nature to view challenges as threats.

Why We React the Way We Do

What are our survival drives?

First, we are programmed to survive as individuals. You must preserve your life before you can do anything else.

Then we are programmed for survival of the species.

To preserve our own life, we must have certain things: We cannot go more than a month or so without food. We need water every few days. And just a few minutes without air can be fatal.

We must also have good health, fitness, and strength to enhance our ability to flee from danger, or to overcome anything or anyone that threatens our life.

To preserve the species, we must find a strong and healthy mate, someone who is attracted to us.

In fact, being socially popular can enhance our individual chances of survival, since other group members can help us fight off danger. Being strong, fit, healthy, and attractive is important to your ancient survival mechanism.

Your ancestors, who survived in the wilderness, were the people with the strongest survival mechanisms. In fact, they were strong and popular people, or they would not have survived in the jungle. You have inherited their strengths: the strong survival drive, and also their physical, mental, emotional, spiritual, and social strength.

If we have this legacy, then why do we sometimes feel so weak, so vulnerable?

Again, the answer is found in the operation of the survival mechanism. It is so strong that it demands that we react to it. In our modern world, our options are different from those in the jungle of long ago.

When an employer is critical, the survival mechanism perceives this as a threat to our ability to obtain the necessities of life: food, shelter, clothing. But a physical attack is no longer appropriate for us. So what do we do? We reassure the survival mechanism by eating, drinking, smoking—ingesting the substances that are vital for individual survival: food (especially high-calorie food), liquids (the favorites are either high-calorie or intoxicating liquids that have the added "advantage" of providing us a brief escape from reality), and air (in the form of cigarettes, which allow us to "see" our breath, thus reassuring us that we are still, indeed, alive).

Take away any of these "security blankets" and both body and mind will react.

When you reduce your calorie intake so your body will begin to live off of its stored reserves (that's fat), it will begin to panic, as if there were a famine, and your mind will recall images of starving children in Ethiopia. You must combat that—not with logic and speeches from your left brain hemisphere but with powerful images impressed on your right brain hemisphere, which you do while at the alpha brain wave level.

There are many other actions that the survival mechanism perceives as a threat to our individual survival, or the survival of the species: The driver who nearly crashes into us in his haste to beat the traffic. The spouse who ignores us, is insensitive, or is inconsiderate and becomes angry. Our children who frighten us so much with their need to grow and mature in their own—often risky—way. And of course, there are our own failures, shortcomings, doubts, and insecurities that plague us all and trigger the survival mechanism. You get the picture.

Gain Control of Your Life

Well, if the traditional "flight or fight" options of our ancestors are no longer appropriate for us, and overeating, drinking, and smoking are so destructive to us, then what other alternatives are available that will satisfy the demands of the survival mechanism, and help us to reach our goals?

There are many alternatives. We'll explore them in a moment. We'll also look at strategies you can use to attack the problem on many levels.

You have already learned several ways to relax and reduce stress, including taking a deep breath and exhaling, and recalling your ideal place of relaxation. You can calm the restless urgings of your survival mechanism with those techniques, and also by practicing the Long Relaxation Exercise and, while at your level, counting your blessings, visualizing goals, and reviewing your plans to achieve those goals.

We'll also outline the programming possibilities of making changes on the physical, mental, emotional, and psychological levels.

We'll look at what it takes to start new habits, the kind of beneficial habits that superstars have, to help them climb to the top and stay there—and to enjoy every minute of it.

You have a great heritage of success. You have, in your genes, the blueprint for strength and popularity. Your ancestors were the successful ones, the ones who had the characteristics necessary for success. If they hadn't, you wouldn't be here.

You'll learn how to use the alpha dimension to reach deep within yourself and get in touch with that inner strength, that strength that you've always known was there, to become as successful and popular as you've always known—deep within—that you could be.

What you are doing here is much more, much stronger, than a simple behavior modification program. You are actually tapping into your strength, your source. You are using your natural strengths and abilities to become the winner you've always known you could be.

Develop Habits That Lead to Success

How can you develop the kind of habits that superstars have? What gives the superstar athlete such great control over their body? What can you learn from those superstars that can help you get the kind of body you want?

Who comes to mind when you think of a great superstar? There are so many men and women who inspire us with their great ability, with their persistence in the face of adversity and discouragement, with their "heart," as announcers and writers like to say, that you can find one or more to use for inspiration.

Remember what we said earlier about habits? Habits are patterns of behavior that are repeated over and over until it becomes automatic, until it becomes easier to do it than not to.

Right now, you may be in the habit of reaching for food when you are a bit nervous, when you are lonely, when you are bored, when you are thinking, when you are working, when you are involved in a relationship with somebody.

It is very simple to program yourself to do something else instead of eating high-calorie foods with no nutritional value.

A superstar athlete might eat a piece of carrot, or celery, or apple, or some such helpful foods, or take a few deep breaths.

A superstar athlete might do some physical exercise instead of eating. A few sit-ups are simple to do and do not require any equipment.

There is something very interesting about exercise: It decreases appetite. That's right, when you get your blood pumping and circulating throughout your body, taking oxygen and nutrients to muscles and brain cells, you get a very satisfied feeling. To burn off fat, you need to get oxygen into your system, and you get oxygen into your body by doing sustained, aerobic-type exercise.

Eating helpful foods, drinking a glass of water, taking several deep breaths, physical exercise—is there something about this that sounds familiar? Of course. These things satisfy our basic survival needs that we discussed earlier: food, drink, breath. And exercise: Exercise involves the use of muscles and increased oxygen demands, such as our ancestors felt when fleeing or fighting.

There is one other thing that a superstar athlete does. He or she practices positive thinking.

What is positive thinking? It is thinking about what you want, rather than what you don't want.

The average person thinks about the taste of the food, and then probably thinks about the weight they will gain.

The superstar athletes, on the other hand, will think about the kind of body they want and the performance they expect from it. You can only hold one thought at a time, so changing your thought from the food and the fat to the desired physique and the performance can make a big difference.

Be sure to do this while you are eating. Never think of being overweight while you are eating. Instead, while eating, always recall the image that you created of yourself at your ideal weight and size. Whenever you pause to recall that image, also recall the special feeling that you had while you were at the alpha level, and this will help activate more alpha production in your brain.

Use the Untapped Power of Your Mind

One big difference between the superstar athlete and the average person, which is very important, is that the superstars are among the 10 percent of humanity who think with both the left and the right brain hemispheres whenever it is appropriate. So when they think of their desired end result and visualize that mental picture of the perfection they are striving for, they are doing so with the right brain hemisphere.

How is this possible? Let me explain:

We all enter the alpha level—very briefly—approximately 30 times every minute. Those brief flashes of alpha last for only microseconds. Since the superstars are accustomed to doing their thinking in alpha, their experience functioning in the alpha dimension allows them to take advantage of these brief alpha encounters, to program themselves.

And since they are accustomed to that special feeling—that mental or emotional feeling—of being at alpha, they can even make those periods last longer. They do not have to close their eyes and relax to get alpha functioning, and to use their right brain hemisphere to think with and to program themselves.

So their positive thinking becomes much more valuable.

To learn to have more alpha functioning the way the superstars do, practice, practice, practice.

There are additional Silva Method programs that can help you develop this kind of full-time alpha functioning. The best of all is the Silva Ultra-Mind ESP System. You can learn more about it in the Resources section of the Appendix.

Graduates of the Silva UltraMind ESP System learn how to stay at alpha even with eyes open, and while physically active. Imagine how it would help you to have the full benefits of alpha functioning while active.

José Silva's Techniques for Reducing Your Weight

Now let's consider some practical techniques you can begin using right away to help you achieve your goal of a trim, fit, healthy, attractive body.

First of all, remember to use some common sense. If you take in more calories than you burn up, if you continue to eat high-calorie foods, lots of sweets, lots of between-meal snacks, and you sit around all day and do not have any physical activity, then you are not very likely to reduce your weight, no matter what you do.

One of the beautiful things about programming yourself at the alpha level is that you will find yourself desiring to modify your behavior so that you are doing the things that will bring you success.

So be aware of your eating and exercise habits. Enter the alpha level, analyze yourself, then program to start some new habits. In the beginning, it may not be easy to develop new habits. That is because you have adapted to your old habits. But persist and you will succeed.

The fact that you're here, the fact that you have already come this far with this program, proves that you have the most important ingredients for success. Remember that you are descended from a long line of survivors. By practicing these techniques, you will put your inherited success traits to work to help you reach your goals. And this is so.

The Easy Way to Exercise

Let's say you want to do some light exercise, so you decide that you will get up an hour earlier, go to a nearby mall, and walk briskly, along with other people who are taking that kind of exercise.

That first morning, it might be pretty easy to get up because you have so much enthusiasm and desire. But how about the next morning? You see, this is a new habit. Your old habit is to remain in bed for another hour. That is what you are comfortable with. Anything we encounter that we are not familiar with triggers the survival mechanism: "Is this something that could be a threat to our survival? Or is this something that could enhance our survival if we capture it?" Either way, the survival mechanism gives us energy. It creates tension with the idea that this tension can propel us into action and enhance our chances of survival.

Well, it's easier to just stay in bed, to stick with the old familiar patterns of behavior, than to deal with this tension created by the survival mechanism.

But once the new pattern of behavior has been repeated enough so that it is now a familiar action, the situation changes.

When you are accustomed to getting up and going to the mall to walk for an hour, then you will not feel comfortable staying in bed for an extra hour. It's true. Even though you are in bed, you will begin to feel uneasy. When you get up and go to the mall, you will feel fine, because you are doing what is familiar to you.

Program New Eating Habits at the Inner Conscious Level

The same with your eating habits: Once you are accustomed to eating foods that are good for you, then you will feel more comfortable eating them than eating foods that make you fat.

To decide which foods are good for you, and which make you fat, check them out at level. When you desire to reduce weight, enter level 1 by the use of the 3 to 1 method and analyze your weight problem. At level 1, mentally mark a big red "No" over every item of food considered to be causing the problem. This way, when you are tempted to eat this food, you will be alerted and can make a conscious choice whether to eat it or not.

You can also use level 1 as a shortcut to establishing new habits. Which would you rather do: Force yourself to perform an activity you are uncomfortable with for several weeks until you get used to it, or program yourself at level 1 to accept it?

Rewrite Your Personal History

The alpha brain wave level is the level of childhood. Children from seven to fourteen years old function more in alpha than in any other range of brain functioning. So when you are functioning at alpha, you are using the part of your brain that you used as a child.

When you program yourself while at the alpha level, it is as though you are a child again, at least as far as the brain is concerned. So if you make mental movies of yourself engaged in certain activities, it is as though you had actually done those things before.

That means that something can become an old habit just by thinking about it, provided you think about it at the alpha level.

Here's another habit you can develop: Program yourself to leave something on your plate, realizing that you do not need all the food you have taken. Program yourself not to eat dessert.

Your natural inclination is to eat when you feel hungry. That is your survival mechanism calling to you. When you begin to reduce weight, your body begins to live off its stored fat. Your body literally begins to consume itself, for survival. Naturally, this triggers your survival mechanism. It becomes very insistent that you ingest food, calories, nutrients. In fact, your body will even slow down its functioning—which you can sense—to conserve as much stored fuel as possible. That's the familiar plateau that we experience a few days after starting a weight loss program.

How can you put this to work for you? Simple: Program yourself that you want to feel hungry. Program yourself to remember that whenever you feel hungry, that means your body is doing exactly what you want it to do: using up stored fuel—using up fat—so that you are becoming leaner, healthier, and sexier, and your weight is coming down. Recall your mental image of the way you want to look. This will motivate you to stick with your plan.

Bodybuilders, who use weights to help them strengthen and enlarge their muscles while reducing body fat to the bare minimum, have a saying: "No pain, no gain." So realize that when you feel hungry, your body is letting you know that you are moving toward your goal. Congratulate yourself, encourage this feeling, and look forward to it. It is excellent feedback that you are winning.

Be sure to eat small, balanced meals every day. It is when we fail to eat a balanced diet that we get headaches, feel sick and irritable, and so forth. It is a very good idea to take a good vitamin supplement to ensure that you are not deficient in any of the nutrients you need to maintain peak health and energy.

An overweight person does not need a lot of calories: some carbohydrates, from foods such as vegetables, fruits, and whole grains; some protein, just a little unsaturated fat, and sufficient vitamins and minerals. Consume these, and you may feel a little hungry—which is what you desire—but you will never feel ill or irritable.

Program all of this at level 1, and it will be easy—even desirable.

Increase Your Motivation and Desire

Now here is one more technique that you can use, and it is a very powerful technique. You can use visualization and imagination at the alpha level to create an image of exactly what you desire.

First, you must set your goals. Remember what we said earlier, about setting goals that you can believe. Belief is very important. Belief is part of faith.

Faith is made up of three elements: desire, belief, and expectancy.

Desire is extremely important. Desire is what drives you toward your goal. It is their powerful desire to avoid failure and to succeed that gives superstar athletes such drive and energy.

You can increase your desire. You increase desire by thinking of all the reasons you have for reaching your goal. That's why earlier I had you get pencil and paper and write down your reasons. Continue to write down reasons you have for reaching your goals, and look at these reasons whenever you need to increase your desire, your motivation, your resolve to succeed.

Who else will benefit when you have a leaner, healthier body? Your family? Your employer? Your friends? The more people who benefit, the stronger your desire to succeed will be.

Motivation is a lot like nutrition: you need it regularly.

Belief is important, because if you do not believe in your goal, in your ability to achieve it, then you will probably quit. That's why it is important to set realistic goals for yourself. Perhaps you desire to reduce 50 pounds. Can you believe it? If not, how about 10 pounds? They say that a journey of a thousand miles begins with a single step. You can take your journey step by step, one step at a time. If you reduce just one pound a week, in a year you will be 50 pounds lighter. Be patient—and also be persistent.

Expectancy is what you do at level 1: You program for your desired end result. And you keep expecting it all the time. Whenever you think of your weight, recall the image of your perfect body.

Actually, at level 1, you create that perfect body. They say that inside every heavy person is a skinny person trying to get out. At level 1, you use your imagination to create that slender, trim, fit, and healthy body. From then on, whenever you think of your weight, visualize—recall—that image you have created. Of course, you may be doing your programming in steps; just remember to visualize—recall—that image you create at level 1.

You may have noticed that I use the word "reduce" rather than "lose" weight. This is part of our positive thinking, what we call mental housecleaning. If you lose something, you usually want to find it and get it back. So let's reduce weight rather than lose it. Also, let's avoid saying we are "giving up" certain foods. Let's focus instead on the positive aspect, on the goal we have, on what we are gaining: that slender, trim, fit, healthy, sexy body.

Look for the Good and Praise It

There's one more thing to say about positive thinking. Some people like to beat themselves up mentally. You don't see superstar athletes doing that. Just think of the superstars you admire. If they make a mistake, they quickly put it out of their mind and come back and perform correctly the next time.

But sometimes a person who has been reducing weight for a couple of weeks decides to binge, to stuff, to pig out. Okay, that's a mistake. Everybody makes mistakes. Nobody is perfect. Nobody.

But this is not failure. You only fail when you give up, when you quit trying. And that's what some people do.

Never give up. Never quit. You can always come back. If you are taking a trip and you make a wrong turn, that's all right; just get back on the right road as soon as possible. It will take you a little longer to get to your destination, but you will still get there.

The key is desire, motivation. You have to keep feeding yourself mentally, just as surely as you must feed yourself physically. Both physically and mentally, you must avoid junk food, and you must consume the highest quality products available. And you must do so regularly. You need motivation and inspiration just as often as you need food. Encourage other people to think the way you do. Hang out with winners and you will develop more winning characteristics. Take advantage of the inspiring workshops and books available from

Silva Method UltraMind. And most importantly, program yourself at level 1 every day—every single day—for success. If you are really serious, program three times a day.

Creating Your New Body at the Alpha Level

In the exercise that follows, you will first enter level 1 with the 3 to 1 method. After the routine-deepening exercises, beneficial statements, and so forth, we will program new information for your benefit.

First, we will review the suggestions we have made to help you change your habits, to control your appetite and reduce your weight. Select the suggestions that you determine at level are appropriate for you at this time, and program yourself to put them into practice.

Then we'll program a special visualization/imagination exercise to help you get the body you want.

To use the visualization technique, you will imagine that you are looking at a full-length mirror. This mirror is slightly above your line of sight, approximately 20 degrees above the horizontal. This is an angle similar to the screen in a movie theater.

The mirror is tall enough so that you can mentally picture yourself full height, and it is three times as wide as it is tall. It is divided into three square sections. One section is directly in front of you, the other sections are to your left.

In the section of the mirror directly in front of you, you will visualize yourself the way you are now. In this section of the mirror, recall what you look like. It may help you to look at yourself in a full-length mirror just prior to doing this exercise, to make it easier for you to recall exactly how your body looks. The more details you can recall, the better.

After you have made a good study of the problem, the way you look now, shift your attention to the second section of the mirror, the section toward your left.

In the second section of the mirror, imagine yourself doing what you need to do to reduce your weight. Imagine your new habit patterns and imagine enjoying them. Mentally picture yourself enjoying eating the foods that you know are good for you. Mentally picture yourself enjoying physical activity that will help you reach and maintain your ideal weight and size. And mentally picture your body beginning to respond the way you want it to.

Then shift your attention to the third section of the mirror, the section farthest to your left. In this section of the mirror, imagine yourself at your ideal weight and size, and imagine your desired weight stamped on one corner of this section of the mirror, and your desired size of clothing stamped on the other corner.

The next time you practice this exercise, use only the second and third sections of the mirror, and visualize—recall—the images you have created of your body responding, and your desired end result: your slender, trim, healthy, attractive body. Whenever you think of your weight, visualize the image you have created of yourself at your ideal weight and size.

Do not go back to the first image again until you have noticed changes taking place in your appearance. At that time, you may go back to the first section of the mirror and alter image number 1 accordingly. Then concentrate on images 2 and 3 until you notice further changes taking place in your body. Remember that you want to spend most of your time focusing on your desired end result. After the first time, always focus on your desired end result.

Small Steps Produce Big Results

You can reach your goal in several steps. For instance, if you decide to reduce just 10 pounds in the first step, then the image in the third section of the mirror, the section farthest to your left, will be of yourself 10 pounds lighter, and this will be indicated in the weight and clothing size you stamp in the corners of the mirror.

After you reach this goal, after you reduce to this weight, then make a new project: In the first section of the mirror, visualize yourself at this new weight that you have achieved, and then imagine yourself in the second section of the mirror, to your left, reducing even further. In the third section of the mirror, farthest to your left, create an image of yourself at the new goal.

In subsequent sessions, use only the second and third sections of the mirror, and whenever you think of your weight, visualize the image you have created of yourself at your ideal weight and size in the third section of the mirror.

The first time you practice this technique, visualize yourself in the first section of the mirror long enough to analyze the problem—to notice details. This might take a minute or two.

Spend more time in the second section of the mirror, the section toward your left, imagining yourself doing what is appropriate to reduce your weight, and your body beginning to respond. You could do this for eight or 10 minutes.

Then in the third section of the mirror, farthest to your left, imagine yourself at your ideal weight and size for two or three minutes.

In the future, visualize—recall—the images you created in the second and third sections of the mirror. Whenever you are eating, visualize the image you created of yourself in the third section of the mirror, farthest to your left, at your ideal weight and size. Visualize your desired weight stamped on one corner of the mirror, and your desired size of clothing stamped on the other corner of the third section of the mirror.

You will soon become very good at doing this programming. And the great part is, you will enjoy it. It will be easy and natural. It will boost your self-confidence and self-esteem as you realize that you are one of the winners, a descendant of a long line of winners, and with a little persistence and the right tools—the Silva tools—you can be a superstar.

How to Proceed

There are a couple of ways you can proceed:

If you remember the instructions, then just enter your level and do it.

Or you can record the script below and let the recording guide you.

When you are ready, find a place where you can make yourself comfortable and not be disturbed for about a half hour and practice the mental exercise.

Keep your eyes closed until you are finished. If you need to open your eyes, open them and make yourself comfortable, then when you are ready, close your eyes and start again at the beginning.

And remember that the greatest discovery you will ever make is the potential of your own mind.

Thank you.

Chapter 8

Silva Superstars' Weight Loss Conditioning

Welcome to the Silva Weight Control Mental Training Exercise.

Before using the exercise, you should have already learned how to enter the alpha level, and by now you should have practiced relaxing physically and mentally at the alpha level at least three times.

You must practice this exercise with your eyes closed, so do not use it while you are driving or engaged in any other activity where you must use your eyesight. Remember that any time you feel tense or nervous and desire to relax, mentally or verbally repeat the word "relax" and you will relax physically and mentally.

Deepening

We will begin this exercise with the 3 to 1 method.

Assume a comfortable position, close your eyes, take a deep breath, and, while exhaling, mentally repeat and visualize the number 3, three times. (pause)

Take another deep breath, and, while exhaling, mentally repeat and visualize the number 2, three times. (pause)

Take another deep breath, and, while exhaling, mentally repeat and visualize the number 1, three times. (pause)

You are now at level 1, the basic plane level that you are learning to use for a purpose, any purpose you desire.

Deepening (routine cycle)

To help you enter a deeper, healthier level of mind, I am going to count from 10 to 1. On every descending number, you will feel yourself going deeper, and you will enter a deeper, healthier level of mind.

10—9—Feel going deeper,

8—7

6—deeper and deeper,

5—4

3—deeper and deeper,

2—1

You are now at a deeper, healthier level of mind, deeper than before.

You may enter a deeper, healthier level of mind by simply relaxing your eyelids. Relax your eyelids. (pause) Feel how relaxed they are. (pause) Allow this feeling of relaxation to flow slowly downward throughout your body, all the way down to your toes. (pause)

It is a wonderful feeling to be deeply relaxed, a very healthy state of being.

To help you enter a deeper, healthier level of mind, I am going to count from 1 to 3. At that moment, you will project yourself mentally to your ideal place of relaxation. I will then stop talking to you, and when you next hear my voice, one hour of time will have elapsed at this level of mind. My voice will not startle you; you will take a deep breath, and, as you exhale, you will relax and go deeper.

1—(pause)—2—(pause)—3. Project yourself mentally to your ideal place of relaxation until you hear my voice again. Relax. (Lecturer: Remain silent for about 30 seconds.)

Relax. (pause) Take a deep breath and, as you exhale, relax and go deeper. (pause)

Rapport

You will continue to listen to my voice; you will continue to follow the instructions at this level of the mind and any other level, including the outer conscious level. This is for your benefit. You desire it, and it is so.

Whenever you mentally or verbally mention the word "relax," all unnecessary movements and activities of your body, brain, and mind will cease immediately, and you will become completely passive and relaxed physically and mentally.

You may bring yourself out of this level or a deeper level than this by counting from 1 to 5. At the count of 5, your eyes will open; you will be wide awake, feeling fine and in perfect health.

Genius Statements

The difference between genius mentality and lay mentality is that geniuses use more of their minds and use them in a special manner.

You are now learning to use more of your mind and to use it in a special manner.

Beneficial Statements

The following are beneficial statements that you may occasionally repeat while at these levels of the mind. Repeat mentally after me.

(Reader: Read slowly.)

My increasing mental faculties are for serving humanity better.

Every day, in every way, I am getting better, better, and better.

Positive thoughts bring me benefits and advantages I desire.

I have full control and complete dominion over my sensing faculties at this level of the mind and any other level, including the outer conscious level. And this is so.

Preventative Statements

The following preventive statements are for your better health. Keep in mind that from now on, I will occasionally be speaking in your place. (Lecturer: Read slowly.)

I will never learn to develop, physically or mentally, mental disorders or psychosomatic or functional ailments or diseases.

I will never learn to develop, physically or mentally, a dependence on drugs or alcohol.

Negative thoughts and negative suggestions have no influence over me at any level of the mind.

I will always maintain a perfectly healthy body and mind.

Mental Projection Statements

Mental Projection statements for success. (Lecturer: Read slowly.)

I am now developing my ability to project my sensing faculties, and to attune my intelligence, to any problem area so as to become aware of any abnormalities, if this is necessary and beneficial for humanity.

I am now beginning to use my ability to project my sensing faculties, and to correct any abnormality I detect.

Negative thoughts and negative suggestions have no influence over me at any level of the mind.

Impression of New Information

We will now impress and program Habit Control, mental techniques you can use to control the eating habit and reduce your weight to your ideal weight.

When you decide to reduce weight, enter level 1 by the use of the 3 to 1 method and analyze your weight problem. At level 1, mentally mark a big red "No" over every item of food considered to be causing the problem.

Program yourself that hunger between meals will vanish by eating a piece of carrot, celery, or apple, or some such helpful foods, or by taking three deep breaths.

Program yourself to leave something on your plate, realizing that you do not need all the food you have taken. Program yourself not to eat dessert.

Use the Mirror Technique. Imagine you are looking at a mirror. This mirror is tall enough so that you can mentally picture yourself full height. It is placed at a height so that you must turn your eyes slightly upward, about 20 degrees, to look at it.

This mirror is three times as wide as it is tall, and it is divided into three square sections, the first one directly in front of you, the other two toward your left. The section of mirror directly in front of you is numbered Section Number 1. The section toward your left is numbered Section Number 2. The section farthest to your left is numbered Section Number 3.

To reduce your weight with the Mirror Technique, enter level 1 with the 3 to 1 method, then imagine that you are looking into the three-section mirror.

Visualize an image of yourself the way you look now, in Section Number 1, directly in front of you, in order to make a good study of the problem. Recall what you look like.

After making a good study of the problem in Section Number 1, direct your attention to the section of the mirror to your left, Section Number 2, and imagine yourself doing what is necessary to correct the problem. Imagine yourself eating foods that will help you reduce your weight. Imagine yourself doing the exercises that will help you reach your goal. While doing this, imagine the desired changes starting to take place. Imagine your body beginning to respond as you continue to reduce toward your ideal weight and size. Imagine yourself enjoying the entire process, and your friends and loved ones admiring you and being inspired by your example.

Next, direct your attention to the section of the mirror farthest to your left, to Section Number 3, and create with your imagination an image of yourself the way you want to be, at your ideal weight and size. Stamp what you want to weigh on one corner of Section Number 3, and the size of dress or suit you want to wear on the other corner of Section Number 3 of the mirror.

In the future, any time you happen to think of your weight, recall and visualize the image you created of yourself in Section Number 3.

In the future, when you notice your body beginning to respond, then at that time go back to image number 1 and alter it accordingly. After that, concentrate on images 2 and 3 until you notice additional changes taking place in your appearance. Then once again update image number 1, and then continue to focus on images 2 and 3.

Whenever you are eating, visualize yourself in Section 3 of the mirror the way you want to look, and visualize your desired weight stamped on one corner and your desired size of clothing stamped on the other corner of Section 3 of the mirror.

Post Effects—Standard

Every time you function at these levels of the mind, you will receive beneficial effects physically and mentally.

You may use these levels of the mind to help yourself, to help your loved ones, to help any human being who needs help, physically and mentally.

You will never use these levels of the mind to harm any human being. If this be your intention, you will not be able to function at these levels of the mind.

You will always use all of your abilities in a constructive, creative manner, to help correct problems. And this is so.

You will continue to take part in constructive and creative activities to make this a better world to live in, so that when we move on, we shall have left behind a better world for those who follow. You will consider the whole of humanity, depending on their ages, as fathers or mothers, brothers or sisters, sons or daughters. You are a superior human being; you have greater understanding, compassion, and patience with others.

Bringout

I will now allow time for you to program by applying your learned techniques. When you are ready, count yourself out of your level with the 1 to 5 method, in perfect health. Take your time.

Chapter 9

The Most Effective Way to Exercise

One of the most valuable additions to any weight control program is . . . exercise.

Now I know some people are thinking, *But isn't this whole program about using your mind to reduce your weight?*

Yes, it is, and after we talk about the benefits of exercising and some of the things I've learned during the 50 years that I've exercised regularly, about how to get more benefit with less work, then I'll show you how to use your mind to get more benefit from your exercise program.

I'll give you a formula that you can use to motivate yourself with your "inner coach," and then program yourself to make exercising easier, more fun, and more effective. Fair enough?

Benefits of Exercise

Now let me tell you about some of the benefits of exercise. For me, it is almost essential. When I'm exercising, I can increase my weight when I want to and can bring it down with no problem at all. Without exercise, it is very difficult.

There are so many other benefits to exercise: It helps to normalize all bodily functions. Exercise gets your heart pumping a little faster and blood flowing through your arteries and veins a little faster—so the heart grows stronger and the circulatory system gets flushed out. Organs and glands are called on even more than normal when you exercise, so they begin to work better. It is the old "use it or lose it" principle.

The digestive processes work better. This is especially true when I do squats—deep knee bends. It is like massaging all of the internal organs. My bowel function improves—bowel movements are more regular, and less difficult.

Exercise decreases appetite. That's right, when you get hungry, go do some exercise and you won't be as hungry. Not because you're tired. I'm not sure that my theory will stand up to strict scientific scrutiny, but here's what I think:

When you exercise, your muscles require fuel. This is true whether you are walking or lifting heavy weights, riding a bike or swimming laps. Some of the stored fuel in your body is released into the bloodstream so that it can be transported to the muscles where it will be used—and since there is plenty of fuel available in your body, you don't feel hungry anymore. Well, I don't know if it is true or not, but it works.

When you are practicing a regular exercise program, you will find that your eating habits improve. Your body stores fuel more efficiently. It craves what it needs for the demands that you are making on it.

Exercise Helps Bring Success in Life

Here's something that wasn't known for a long, long time—and even today not everybody knows: Exercise is extremely important for success in every area of life—not just health, but also relationships, business, and personal development.

Growing up in the newspaper business, as a reporter, covering activities of the business community, politics, police beat, and all the rest, I got to know a lot of people "at the top." One of the things that I learned long ago is that most of them exercise so they will have the energy and the good health that is necessary to do all the work that is required in order to achieve so much success. Heads of corporations, high-level politicians, university presidents—these are some of the people I knew who exercised regularly, even though few people outside of their closest friends and associates knew it.

Of course, exercise provides many health benefits. A friend of mine, a little over 40 years of age, just got the reports of her lab tests: borderline osteoporosis—weak bones; borderline diabetes; and high blood pressure.

Every one of those conditions will benefit from exercise.

Exercise will strengthen your bones, just as it will strengthen your skeletal muscles, your heart and lungs, your circulatory system, your organs and glands, your digestive system, and even your brain. Okay, maybe I'm stretching it a little bit, but I believe that when you get more blood flowing and carrying more oxygen, your brain is bound to benefit too.

My friend mentioned to her doctor what I had said about exercising being good for all three of her medical problems. He said that was absolutely true, that he didn't bother mentioning it because he figured that nowadays, everybody knows the value of exercise, so if they're not exercising it's because they just don't want to.

That brings up two valuable points:

First, always consult with your doctor before starting any exercise program. And when you are dealing with health problems—as my friend is—then make sure you keep your doctor advised of what you experience once you begin to exercise. Let your doctor help you evaluate whatever changes take place—good or bad. Your doctor can help you make sure that you make the best possible progress in improving your medical condition.

The second point is, a lot of people still just don't want to exercise. I know that you have good reasons for not exercising—too many other responsibilities to your family and your job, no place to exercise, no money for the right exercise clothing, too cold, too hot, too dark, too light. You don't have to tell me . . . because I've heard every excuse there is. In fact, I've used every excuse there is to keep from having to exercise!

No Excuses for Not Exercising

Even if you have health problems, you can still exercise. If you're flat on your back in a hospital bed, you can still grab the bar up above you and pull on it! You can always do something.

In 1995 a man named Raymond Horn from Houston, Texas, sent us a beautiful testimonial, including his picture. We used his story in the Silva Method Newsletter, and also in our *Think and Grow Fit* book, published by Career Press. Here is what he told us:

"In 1957 I spent 40 days and nights in a hospital with bleeding ulcers. Doctors removed half of my stomach.

"I was determined not to be sick again.

"I started running, using the Silva Method to convince myself I could run.

"Then," he continued, "I decided to run a marathon—at 63 years of age—by using Silva.

"I ran a 26.2 mile marathon in Honolulu, Hawaii, in 1982. Since that time I have run 16 marathons in a row.

"I give 100 percent of the credit to using the Silva Method.

"I believe if I could run a marathon, you can too. I am 79 years of age.

"You need to train for six months . . . and use the Silva Method every day.

"I was never considered an athlete in high school or college," he added at the end.

Raymond Horn is a certified public accountant in Houston. He ran the 1991 Honolulu Marathon in 6 hours, 12 minutes, and finished seventh out of 14 males aged 75 to 79.

So your excuses are not going to work with me. I didn't let my excuses let me off the hook when I tried to use them, so I'm sure not going to accept any excuses from you. In fact, I'll tell you how I overcame my excuses, my laziness, my lack of athletic ability, and all the other reasons for not exercising. I'm kind of an expert at overcoming excuses . . . and doing what I should be doing.

You see, I've had some great teachers through the years, ever since I began exercising at the age of five. I didn't have much of a choice—I had polio when I was five, and it was exercise that restored enough function to my crippled legs so that I could learn to walk again.

As far as I'm concerned, Dr. Robert L. Bennett is the smartest man who ever lived—and the most practical. He made it easy for you to do the right thing. When I went to him as a teenager in the 1950s and asked him to give me an exercise routine, I had learned by then that if I didn't exercise, I experienced pain in my legs, and just pain didn't feel very good.

"I could give you a calisthenics routine," he told me, "but nobody does calisthenics, and you wouldn't do them for very long either."

I had to admit that he was right. So he told me to do this: "Go to any hardware store," he said, "any buy a spring or a weight system, and follow the instructions."

That was it. The greatest doctor in the world. The man who treated more polio patients than anybody else, who helped us learn to walk again, the director of the world-famous polio rehab facility at Warm Springs, Georgia—where President Roosevelt died—told me to buy any kind of exercise equipment at a hardware store and just follow the instructions.

He understood a couple of things very well: First, lifting weights—which is still an Olympic sport—is a whole lot more interesting than doing calisthenics, and if it was interesting, I would keep doing it. Second, if I selected something that appealed to me, I'd be much more likely to keep doing it than if he assigned me to do the exact same thing. We all like to choose, to be in control, don't we?

So here is my first bit of advice: Don't let somebody else decide what you should do. Don't follow some routine just because a celebrity says it is good. Instead, find what you like, find what interests you, and what works best for you. Then you'll stick with it.

How Habits Can Help You

Exercise is a habit, or it should be. And you know what a habit is: It is something that you are accustomed to doing, that you have done so often, for so long, that it is now easier to do it than not to.

In the beginning, exercise is not a habit. So you have to remind yourself to do it. You have to tell yourself to do it. You have to persuade yourself to do it. I'll get into motivation techniques a little later. Guilt is a technique that works very well for me. I'll explain how in a moment. For now, realize that you will have to remember to do it in the beginning, until you are so accustomed to exercising that you don't feel right when you don't do it. That is when it has become a habit.

But exercise is a habit that is very easy to break. That's unfortunate, isn't it? So guard against the danger of "breaking" the exercise habit. Do whatever you have to do keep this habit.

Here's something I didn't know for a long, long time about exercise. If you follow a very simple schedule that I will give you in just a moment, it will be easy to make it a lifetime habit.

Strategies to Help Create New Habits

Here is the problem that most people have: They start to exercise and they keep on exercising and exercising, day after day, week after week, until it becomes work. What might have been fun in the beginning becomes work. You can develop a real aversion to just about anything if you continue to overdo it. So follow these guidelines:

First, exercise builds you up; work wears you down. It is normal to feel tired immediately after a workout, but an hour or so later, you should feel relaxed and good.

If you continue to feel tired and drained the rest of the day, then you didn't do exercise—you did work! Work wears you down. As somebody said, you know work is a bad thing when they have to pay people to do it! My point is, you want to do enough to stimulate your body to perform at a higher level, not tear it down and wear it out with overwork.

Yes, I know the old saying, "No pain, no gain." Just remember this: If you are not making enough progress through your exercise, then do less. That's right, try doing less. You have to give your body time for recovery, to rebuild the tissues that you have broken down through exercise, and to add a little bit more, to overcompensate so that you have some reserve to do even more the next time.

Here's one more guideline to keep you from becoming stale and burned out: After exercising for six weeks, take a week off. That's a schedule that works out best for most people. You can experiment with it—maybe you'll want to take a week off after five weeks. Or you might even want to go longer than six weeks.

Take that week off even if you don't want to. In fact, that's ideal—you definitely don't want to keep working out until you are burned out physically, mentally, and emotionally. I used to do that. I'd work out for three months and be so burned out that I'd quit for six months. By then my body would be demanding that I help it out by exercising it, so I'd start again, work really hard for three or four months, then stop again for six months. Or sometimes longer. That's no good.

Stop when you still feel good, before you get burned out, and take the full week off. That's one of those times that I use guilt to motivate me.

If you are training three times a week, and you skip three workouts, that means that you do your final workout on a Friday, skip the entire next week—skip workouts on Monday, Wednesday, and Friday—and don't do your next workout until the following Monday, a full 10 days without a workout. Believe me, by that time I am feeling guilty about not working out and am eager to get back to it.

Remember: On average, take one week off every six weeks.

Have fun with your exercise too. Do things you enjoy. Vary what you do. I work sometimes with barbells, other times with dumbbells. I walk, I run, I swim, and I love to ride my bicycle. Variety keeps you fresh. It also works different parts of your body, different muscles, and works them from different angles. This gives you great overall conditioning.

Do What Is Appropriate for Your Body Type

There are a lot of different body types, and different body types require different training routines. And you cannot change your body type . . . so learn to accept it.

All you need to do is to look around you to see that some people are big, some are small, and other people fall somewhere in between.

My friend Vera Christensen, a pioneer in women's physique training, has operated health clubs and trained thousands of women and men since the early 1960s, and she was the women's editor of *Strength and Health* magazine for more than 30 years. "Everybody has different bone structure," she says. "Any good instructor can look at you and know what kind of training you need."

How can you determine for yourself what your training needs are?

Vera says, "Most people know what kind of bodies they have. Women almost always know. When they buy clothes, they can tell. If the top part of their body is too small and the bottom part too big for the clothes, then they know what kind of body they have."

It's usually pretty easy to determine your body type: Take your clothes off and look in a mirror.

Vera Christensen has people send her photographs of their bodies, both front and side views, so that she can evaluate them and prescribe specific training routines for them.

Another way is to go to a good trainer or coach and ask for a complete evaluation. Dr. William Sheldon noted that any coach who cannot quickly spot relatively small variations in physique will not be a successful coach, because there are such different training methods required for different physiques.

Dr. Sheldon noted that men generally fall into three basic categories, which he wrote about in his book *Varieties of Human Physique*:

Ectomorphs are the very small-boned people, slender, who find it difficult to gain weight. Barney Fife on the old Andy Griffith television show is a good example.

Mesomorphs are people with a great athletic build. They are well-proportioned and look like good athletes.

Endomorphs are the big boys—large bones, big stomach, the kind who play offensive lineman on the football team, the kind who become professional wrestlers.

Ectomorphs need to be very careful not to overtrain. Workouts should not be longer than an hour, and they should not train on consecutive days. They need at least one full day of rest between workouts, often more. If you are an ectomorph and you aren't making much progress, then do less. Do quality exercises—don't waste time with little dumbbells, for instance; do presses and squats. Keep your sessions short, so you don't tire yourself out. And take plenty of rest time before your next workout.

Mesomorphs and endomorphs can handle heavier routines. But the advice still holds—if you are not making enough progress by increasing your workouts, try decreasing them. Give your body time to recover from the workout, and some more time to overcompensate and build up some reserves so that you can handle an even heavier load next time. If you allow only enough time to barely recover from a workout, and not enough time for the body to overcompensate, then you won't grow stronger.

Vera Christensen notes that the following body types are the most common in women:

Number 1. Small top, big bottom. They usually need calf work.

Number 2. Big top and middle (waist), and small bottom. Both hips and legs are small and need more development.

Number 2A. This variation of the second type is the same except that they have rugged, muscular legs. They are usually shorter, but not always. While they can be excellent athletes, they are not good candidates for beauty contests.

Number 3. Long legs and a big upper hip area. The top portion of their body is usually quite nice. They often have flat feet, which tends to cause them to slump and can lead to back problems.

Men are similar, she said. Some of the most common male physiques are:

1. Broad shoulders, slim hips and legs.
2. Narrow shoulders, broader hips and waist, medium to thin legs.
3. Stocky all over, large-boned.

"I don't see too many really symmetrical women," Vera said. "There is a slightly higher percentage of symmetrical men than women."

With those guidelines in mind, and with the recommendations of your coach or trainer, you can enter your level, and at alpha determine the best routine for you.

There is a very easy way to tell if you have come up with the correct answer at your level—at the alpha level: Put your ideas to the test, and observe the results that you get.

If you feel, at your level, that you are not training as hard as you should, then train harder and observe the results that you get. If you make progress, you were correct. If not, then enter your level and try again.

If you feel, at your level, that you should take an extra day's rest between workouts, then do so, and observe your results. If you seem to have more energy and you work harder, then you were correct.

Whether you are right or wrong at your level, you can use this information to establish "points of reference." In other words, you learn what works and what doesn't. You do the same thing in athletics: When something works, you know to keep practicing and get better at it. If it doesn't work, then avoid it.

Continue to use this kind of "trial and error" method at your level, and you will soon learn how to be a superstar at the mental game.

5 Essential Elements of an Exercise Program

There are five essential elements in an exercise routine:

1. Stretching and flexibility. Children are flexible . . . old people are not. When you can't move anymore, you're dead. Get the idea? Always stretch and limber up, even if you do nothing else.
2. Resistance—a little more than usual, and your body will say, "Okay, this person is going to lift 50 pounds, so I will add a little reserve strength so if they try 60, we can handle it." You can lift dumbbells. You can use machines. You can lift a can of pork and beans, a milk jug with water (which makes it easy to vary the weight).
3. Endurance—breathe a little heavier than normal. Walk. Ride a bike. Jog. Swim. Dance—fast dancing or aerobic dancing.

4. Athletic movements for coordination, such as dance, aerobics, etc.
5 Rest, relaxation, and recovery.

Tips to Motivate Yourself

Now I promised to tell you how I have motivated myself to continue to exercise for more than 50 years. I use every trick I can think of: I think of benefits, of course; I make bargains with myself; I use guilt—anything I can think of.

Sometimes I'll tell myself that I really need to clean up around the house. I don't like to do that, so instead I'll exercise. Then I don't feel guilty about not cleaning the house.

Here is something that has worked well for me time and time again. I'll get home in the evening and it is a workout day, but I really don't want to face a bar loaded with 200 pounds of weights, not after the day I just had. So I'll use guilt or bargains with myself or whatever I can to persuade myself that I should go ahead and do something.

What I'll often do is to decide that I will at least keep the routine going, even though I won't actually lift any weights. I'll just put on my workout gear and tape my feet, and that way I will have done something to keep the habit going. Remember that the exercise habit is an easy habit to break, so it is important to guard against breaking it.

After I tape up my feet and put on my exercise gear, it seems a shame to let it go completely to waste, doesn't it? Well, we know how important stretching is. And it always makes you feel good. Never force your stretching; you can hurt yourself if you do. Just relax into it. That's easy enough. So I do my stretching and flexibility work. No problem. Now I can go relax in front of the television and munch on some apple, carrot, or other such healthy food.

Except . . . well, you know what . . . that stretching got my muscles loosened up, got my blood flowing a little more freely, it seems like. In fact, the old "habit" is kicking in. I've gone that far, and the next part of the habit is to take the empty bar—an Olympic weightlifting bar weighs 35 pounds—and I'll just do some warmup movements with it. Lift it from the floor to overhead, up and down, several times. Just go through the motions. No weight, no strain, no effort, no problem.

Well, you know what happens next: I don't want to waste a perfectly good warmup. I mean, changing clothes, stretching out, warming up . . . I might as well put the light weights on the bar and do a few warmup lifts, and then it is straight to the TV.

Of course, you know what happens next: The body is all prepared and ready to pump some heavy iron. So that's what I do.

In fact, some of my very best workouts have come on those days when I was convinced that all I was going to do was to put on my workout gear and go watch television! I've set some personal records on those days.

Small steps make it seem easy. Program to reduce your weight one pound a week—that's easy and believable. Just take things one step at a time, knowing that you can stop any time you wish. But when it's a habit—when you've gotten the "exercise habit"—you'll find that the habit will push you on and you will be grateful.

Do It Mentally First

Okay, we've talked long enough. Now it is time to take some action. It's time to exercise. So let's get started—we'll start the easiest way there is:

Just relax, enter your level, and daydream your way through a complete exercise session.

Then you'll be all fired up and ready to get your body involved too, and you'll have a wonderful workout.

In the mental exercise that follows, we'll enter level, do some deepening, and then program.

First we'll program for motivation. Here's how:

Increase Your Desire

To prepare yourself mentally for a workout, enter the alpha level and review your reasons for working out: You want to look better, feel better, have more energy to carry out your daily activities, and be healthier. Mentally picture yourself the way you want to be. This will motivate you.

For even more motivation, remain at your level and think about how somebody else will benefit from your increased fitness level. Perhaps a family member or friend will be happier when you reach your goals. Perhaps you will perform better work on your job, and your employer will benefit. In fact, think of as many people as you can who will benefit. Your increased health and fitness can serve as an inspiration to others.

The more people who will benefit, the more desire you will have.

Then when you get up to go do your workout . . . you will have a fabulous workout!

Mental Rehearsal

Before you come out of level, you can rehearse the routine mentally.

After you finish the motivation, then mentally go through your entire workout routine. Recall how you feel when you begin. Recall all the things you do, the moves you make, and imagine yourself doing them better than ever before.

Recall how you feel one-quarter of the way into the workout, halfway through, three-quarters of the way through, and as you finish. Rehearse it all mentally, and keep in mind the benefits to you and to others.

Then when you are done, go have a wonderful workout!

You know you want to do it. You know you'll look better, feel better, be healthier, be more resistant to colds and flu and other illnesses.

Do it for your loved ones. They want you to be around for a long time, healthy and fit and active and not a burden to them, but instead a person who will continue to contribute and enrich their lives and be an inspiration to them.

No more excuses. Remember: I've heard them all, and I haven't heard one yet that's acceptable. So go put your exercise clothes on, then make yourself comfortable, enter your level, motivate yourself from within by recalling all the reasons and benefits of getting into great shape and staying that way, rehearse your whole workout mentally, and then go do it and watch the fabulous results you get.

Are you ready? Okay, then . . . let's do it!

Chapter 10

Mental Rehearsal Conditioning Cycle

This is the Mental Rehearsal exercise in the Silva Star Athlete program, to help you achieve your training and athletic goals and become a superstar.

Before using this exercise, you should have already learned how to enter the alpha level, and by now you should have practiced relaxing physically and mentally at the alpha level for at least two hours. You can do this by listening to a recording of the Silva Centering Exercise at least four times and practicing as you are directed.

While learning, you should keep your eyes closed. Therefore, you should not do this while you are driving or engaged in any other activity where you must use your eyesight.

Remember that any time you feel tense or nervous and desire to relax, mentally or verbally repeat the word "relax" and you will relax physically and mentally.

This mental exercise is based on material originally copyrighted by José Silva of Laredo, Texas, in 1969. New material is copyrighted 2026 by José Silva.

You can record this mental exercise and play it back, or you can have somebody read it to you, or you can memorize the steps and do it on your own.

Let your results guide you: When you make progress, keep doing what you are doing. If not, try something different. You can change your routine, change your attitude, try practicing at a different time—do whatever works best for you.

Here is the script, exactly the way we present it in our Silva Star Athlete workshops.

Silva Star Athlete Mental Rehearsal Exercise

We will begin this exercise with the 3 to 1 method.

Assume a comfortable position, close your eyes, take a deep breath and, while exhaling, mentally repeat and visualize the number 3 three times. (pause)

Take another deep breath and, while exhaling, mentally repeat and visualize the number 2 three times. (pause)

Take another deep breath and, while exhaling, mentally repeat and visualize the number 1 three times. (pause)

You are now at level 1, the basic plane level that you are able to use for a purpose, any purpose you desire.

To help you enter a deeper, healthier level of mind, I am going to count from 10 to 1. On each descending number, you will feel yourself going deeper and you will enter a deeper, healthier level of mind.

10—9 Feel going deeper,
8—7
6—deeper and deeper,
5—4
3—deeper and deeper,
2—1

You are now at a deeper, healthier level of mind, deeper than before.

You may enter a deeper, healthier level of mind by simply relaxing your eyelids. Relax your eyelids. (pause) Feel how relaxed they are. (pause) Allow this feeling of relaxation to flow slowly downward throughout your body, all the way down to your toes. (pause). It is a wonderful feeling to be deeply relaxed, a very healthy state of being.

To help you enter a deeper, healthier level of mind, I am going to count from 1 to 3. At that moment, you will project yourself mentally to your ideal place of relaxation. I will then stop talking to you, and when you next hear my voice, one hour of time will have elapsed at this level of mind. My voice will not startle you; you will take a deep breath, relax, and go deeper.

1—(pause)—2—(pause)—3. Project yourself mentally to your ideal place of relaxation until you hear my voice again. Relax. (Reader: Remain silent for about 30 seconds.)

Relax. (pause) Take a deep breath and, as you exhale, relax and go deeper. (pause)

You will continue to listen to my voice; you will continue to follow the instructions at this level of the mind and any other level, including the outer conscious level. This is for your benefit; you desire it, and it is so.

Whenever you mentally or verbally mention the word "relax," all unnecessary movements and activities of your body, brain, and mind will cease immediately, and you will become completely passive and relaxed physically and mentally.

I may bring you out of this level or a deeper level than this by counting to you from 1 to 5. At the count of 5, your eyes will open; you will be wide awake, feeling fine and in perfect health.

The difference between genius mentality and lay mentality is that geniuses use more of their minds and use them in a special manner.

You are now learning to use more of your mind and to use it in a special manner.

The following are beneficial statements that you may occasionally repeat while at these levels of the mind. Repeat mentally after me. (Reader: Read slowly.)

My increasing ability to concentrate helps me perform better, build greater strength and fitness, and develop a better physique.

My increasing health, strength, and fitness are to be used to produce better work and to help correct problems.

My increasing health, strength, and fitness enable me to cope with any kind of task, whatever it might be, and help me to deal with any emergency.

My increasing vitality, energy, and talents are for serving humanity better.

Every day, in every way, I am getting better, better, and better.

Day by day I am growing stronger and healthier, and developing a better physique, so that I may serve as a model for others.

I always maintain a positive attitude because positive thoughts bring me benefits and advantages I desire.

I have full control and complete dominion over my sensing faculties and my energies at this level of the mind and any other level, including the outer conscious level. And this is so.

The following preventive statements are for your better health. Keep in mind that from now on, I will occasionally be speaking in your place. (Reader: Read slowly.)

I will never learn to develop, physically or mentally, mental disorders or psychosomatic or functional ailments or diseases.

I will never learn to develop, physically or mentally, a dependence on drugs or alcohol.

Negative thoughts and negative suggestions have no influence over me at any level of the mind.

I will always maintain a perfectly healthy body and mind.

Mental Projection statements for success. (Lecturer: Read slowly.)

I am now developing my ability to project my sensing faculties, and to attune my intelligence, to any problem area so as to become aware of any abnormalities, if this is necessary and beneficial for humanity.

I am now beginning to use my ability to project my sensing faculties, and to correct any abnormality I detect.

Negative thoughts and negative suggestions have no influence over me at any level of the mind.

Impression of New Information—Programming

We will now impress information for your benefit, programming the Mental Rehearsal Technique, a formula-type technique that you can use to help you gain more benefits from your exercise.

First we'll program for motivation.

To prepare yourself mentally for a workout, enter the alpha level and review your reasons for working out: You want to look better, feel better, have more energy to carry out your daily activities, and be healthier. Mentally picture yourself the way you want to be. This will motivate you.

For even more motivation, remain at your level and think about how somebody else will benefit from your increased fitness level. Perhaps a family member or friend will be happier when you reach your goals.

Perhaps you will perform better work on your job, and your employer will benefit. In fact, think of as many people as you can who will benefit. Your increased health and fitness can serve as an inspiration to others. The more people who will benefit, the more desire you will have. Then when you get up to go do your workout, you will have a fabulous workout!

Mental Rehearsal Practice

After you finish the motivation, then mentally go through your entire workout routine. To do this, you will first project yourself mentally to be at the place where you exercise. Notice your surroundings. (pause)

Once you have projected yourself mentally to the place where you exercise, imagine yourself performing the way you desire. Imagine yourself improving and reaching your goals.

Notice how you feel as you make each movement. Imagine the feeling of your body responding and becoming stronger, more flexible, and more fit.

I will now allow you time to practice your learned techniques. When you hear my voice again, you will relax even more.

(Reader: Pause about one minute.)

Relax. (pause) Take a deep breath and, as you exhale, relax and go deeper.

Programming for Success

In order to make strong impressions of the special feeling of success, whenever you have a success, when you notice that the desired changes are taking place in your body, then as soon as possible, enter level 1. While at level 1, review the things that you did that led to this success, and recall how you felt when you were successful. This will help you to be even more successful in the future. (Pause)

POST EFFECTS

In your next session you will again enter level 1, and you will enter a deeper, healthier level of mind faster and easier than this time.

Every time you function at these levels of the mind, you will receive beneficial effects physically and mentally.

You may use these levels of the mind to help yourself, physically and mentally.

You may use these levels of the mind to help your loved ones, physically and mentally.

You may use these levels of the mind to help any human being who needs help, physically and mentally.

You will never use these levels of the mind to harm any human being; if this be your intention, you will not be able to function within these levels of the mind.

You will always use these levels of the mind in a constructive, creative manner for all that is good, honest, pure, clean, and positive. And this is so.

You will continue to strive to take part in constructive and creative activities to make this a better world to live in, so that when we move on, we shall have left behind a better world for those who follow. You will consider the whole of humanity, depending on their ages, as fathers or mothers, brothers or sisters, sons or daughters. You are a superior human being; you have greater understanding, compassion, and patience with others.

BRINGOUT

In a moment I am going to count from 1 to 5. At that moment, you will open your eyes, be wide awake, feeling fine and in perfect health, feeling better than before. You will have no ill effects whatsoever in your head, no headache; no ill effects whatsoever in your hearing, no buzzing in your ears; no ill effects whatsoever in your vision and eyesight; vision, eyesight, and hearing improve every time you function at these levels of mind.

1—2—coming out slowly now.

3—at the count of 5, you will open your eyes, be wide awake, feeling fine and in perfect health, feeling better than before, feeling the way you feel when you have slept the right amount of revitalizing, refreshing, relaxing, healthy sleep.

4—5 eyes open, wide awake, feeling fine and in perfect health, feeling better than before.

Chapter 11

Mental Video for Habits

Here is a bonus technique, developed by José Silva in 1997, that you can use to help you make better decisions about anything—making or breaking habits, health decisions, family decisions, business decisions.

He named it the MentalVideo Technique.

It is similar to the 3-Mirrors Technique that he developed back in the 1960s, but instead of creating scenes for programming yourself, you are going to create mental scenes to program and solve problems for the greater good.

What is the MentalVideo?

It is a scientific way to pray for verifiable guidance and help from higher intelligence.

What is higher intelligence? It is what some people refer to as God or Jehovah or Allah or The

Almighty or Brahman or Yahweh or many other names.

José Silva had a unique way of looking at it.

"The Universe has billions of galaxies. Our galaxy, which is considered a baby galaxy compared to others, has millions of solar systems. In order to oversee the whole universe it is necessary to have a hierarchy of God," he explained.

"Common sense indicates that God must have billions of helpers. Some call these helpers angels, archangels, and seraphs; others call them guides, and so forth.

"Everyone has a personal representative; we refer to your representative as your Tutor.

"The Tutor is the spiritual guide that resides in the spiritual, subjective dimension (the other side) and is connected to the hierarchy of God to help you solve problems when you are doing the right thing. Your Tutor serves as your personal God."

You Are Special Too

We are all part of this management system. Indications are that we were sent here to planet Earth with a job to do. That job is to correct problems, improve living conditions, and convert the planet into a paragraph.

In order to do our job, we have been given dominion over the planet. We are the highest biological life form on the planet; we have been assigned a superior position and have been given dominion over the planet.

That makes you and everybody else on planet Earth part of the management team that we refer to as higher intelligence.

Business organizations and governments have hierarchical systems. You don't call the mayor to come fix a pothole in the street in front of your house. There is somebody else you can call, and they will send a road repair crew to make the repairs.

We are the "boots on the ground" who are assigned to do the physical work here on planet Earth.

Laws of Programming

There are two important aspects to this technique. One is creating the scenes and images that you will deliver to your tutor.

The other involves attitude and proper motivation. For this, he created something else to be included with this technique, what he called the "Laws of Programming."

The following laws are to be considered when programming:

- You should do to others only what you like others to do to you.
- The solution must help to make this planet a better place to live.
- It must be the best for everybody concerned.
- It must help at least two or more persons.
- It must be within the possibility area.

If we are a part of the human family on planet Earth, then isn't the smart thing to help—not hurt—our family?

When humanity does well, we all do well. A rising tide lifts all ships.

The MentalVideo Technique

This is not an alternative or a replacement for the self-improvement techniques covered earlier in this book.

The MentalVideo is intended to be used in two circumstances:

1. Use it when you reach a sticking point and you do not know what to do next. Present the MentalVideo to higher intelligence—your "tutor"—with the

attitude that you need help to finish the job you are working on.

2. You can also use it to let higher intelligence know what you are working on, what your plans are, and you will continue unless higher intelligence has a better idea.

How do you know if you receive guidance from higher intelligence? Through "coincidences."

If you wish, you can enter your level and "install" this program into your brain as you did the previous techniques, or you can just go ahead and use it.

The MentalVideo Formula:

Whenever you need to solve a problem, make a decision, or obtain guidance with the MentalVideo Technique, proceed in the following manner:

At beta, with your eyes open, mentally create, with visualization, a MentalVideo of a problem, or the existing situation. Include everything that belongs to the animate matter kingdom. Animate matter means everything that contains life.

After you have completed the MentalVideo of the problem, use visualization to review it at beta, with your eyes closed.

Later, when you are in bed and ready to go to sleep, go to your center with the 3 to 1 method. Once you are at your center, review the MentalVideo that you created of the problem, or the existing situation, when you were at the beta level.

After you have reviewed the problem, mentally convert the problem into a project. Then create, with imagination, a MentalVideo of the solution.

The MentalVideo of the solution should contain a step-by-step procedure of how you desire the project to be resolved.

After both of the MentalVideos have been completed, go to sleep with the intention of delivering the MentalVideos to your tutor while you sleep. Take for granted that the delivery will be made.

During the next three days, look for indications that point to the solution. Every time you think of the project, think of the solution that you created in the MentalVideo, in a past tense sense.

Appendix A

Alternative Way to Find the Alpha Level

(Note: It is not necessary to do this if you are learning by listening to a recording of the Centering Exercise or having someone read it to you as you learned in Chapter 6.)

I will give you a simple way to relax, and you will do better and better at this as you practice.

I will also give you a beneficial statement to help you.

This is how you train your mind. You relax, lower your brain frequency to the alpha level, and practice using imagination and visualization.

Because you cannot read this book and relax simultaneously, it is necessary that you read the instructions first, so that you can put the book down, close your eyes, and follow them.

Here they are:

1. Sit comfortably in a chair and close your eyes. Any position that is comfortable is a good position.
2. Take a deep breath, and, as you exhale, relax your body.
3. Count backward slowly from 50 to 1.
4. Daydream about some peaceful place you know.
5. Say to yourself mentally, "Every day, in every way, I am getting better, better, and better."
6. Remind yourself mentally that when you open your eyes at the count of 5, you will feel wide awake, better than before. When you reach the count of 3, repeat this, and when you open your eyes, repeat it ("I am wide awake, feeling better than before").

You already know steps one and two. You do them daily when you get home in the evening. Add a countdown, a peaceful scene, and a beneficial statement to help you become better and better, and you are ready for a final count-out.

Read the instructions once more. Then put the book down and do it.

Learning to Function Consciously at the Alpha Level

As stated previously, you learn to enter the alpha level and function there with just one day of training when you attend the Silva UltraMind ESP Systems live training programs. You can use the audio recordings to learn to enter the alpha level within a few days with either a Silva home-study program or the free lessons at the SilvaNow.com website. You can also record the Silva Centering Exercise in Chapter 6 and listen to it, or have someone read it to you.

If you have already learned to enter the alpha level by one of those methods, you can skip the following instructions for practicing countdown-deepening exercises for the next 40 days.

If not, then follow these instructions from José Silva:

When you enter sleep, you enter alpha. But you quickly go right through alpha to the deeper levels of theta and delta.

Throughout the night, your brain moves back and forth through alpha, theta, and delta, like the ebb and flow of the tide. These cycles last about 90 minutes.

In the morning, as you exit sleep, you come out through alpha, back into the faster beta frequencies that are associated with the outer conscious levels.

Some authors advise that as you go to sleep at night, you think about your goals. That way, you get a little bit of alpha time for programming. The only trouble is, you have a tendency to fall asleep.

For now, I just want you to practice a simple exercise that will help you learn to enter and stay at the alpha level. Then, in 40 days, you will be ready to begin your programming.

In the meantime, I will give you some additional tasks that you can perform at the beta level that will help you prepare yourself so that you will be able to program more effectively at the alpha level when you are ready at the completion of the 40 days.

Your First Assignment

If you are using the Silva Centering Exercise (also known as the Long Relaxation Exercise) on the SilvaNow.com website to enter the alpha level, then you can skip the information that follows.

If you do not want to use the recording of the Silva Centering Exercise, and you have not attended a Silva seminar or used one of our home-study courses to learn to enter the alpha level, then you will need to follow the instructions here to learn to enter the alpha level on your own.

Here is your alpha exercise:

Practice this exercise in the morning when you first wake up. Since your brain is starting to shift from alpha to beta when you first wake up, you will not have a tendency to fall asleep when you enter alpha.

Here Are the Steps to Take

1. When you awake tomorrow morning, go to the bathroom if you have to, then go back to bed. Set your alarm clock to ring in 15 minutes, just in case you do fall asleep again.
2. Close your eyes and turn them slightly upward toward your eyebrows (about 20 degrees relative to your face). Research shows that this produces more alpha brainwave activity.
3. Count backward slowly from 100 to 1. Do this silently; that is, do it mentally to

yourself. Wait about one second between numbers.

4. When you reach the count of 1, hold a mental picture of yourself as a success. An easy way to do this is to recall the most recent time when you were 100 percent successful. Recall the setting, where you were, and what the scene looked like; recall what you did; and recall what you felt like.
5. Repeat mentally, "Every day in every way I am getting better, better, and better."
6. Then say to yourself, "I am going to count from 1 to 5; when I reach the count of 5, I will open my eyes, feeling fine and in perfect health, feeling better than before."
7. Begin to count. When you reach 3, repeat, "When I reach the count of 5, I will open my eyes, feeling fine and in perfect health, feeling better than before, feeling as though I have slept the right amount of revitalizing, refreshing, relaxing, healthy, wonderful sleep."
8. Continue your count to 4 and 5. At the count of 5, open your eyes and tell yourself mentally, "I am wide awake, feeling fine and in perfect health, feeling better than before. And this is so."

These Eight Steps Are Really Only Three

Go over each of these eight steps so that you understand the purpose while at the same time become more familiar with the sequence.

1. The mind cannot relax deeply if the body is not relaxed. It is better to go to the bathroom and permit your body to enjoy full comfort. Also, when you first awake, you may not be fully awake. Going to the bathroom ensures your being fully awake. But in case you are still not awake enough to stay awake, set your alarm clock to ring in 15 minutes so you do not risk being late on your daily schedule. Sit in a comfortable position.
2. Research has shown that when a person turns their eyes up about 20 degrees, it triggers more alpha rhythm in the brain and also causes more right-brain activity. Later, when we do our mental picturing, it will be with your eyes turned upward at this angle. Meanwhile, it is a simple way to encourage alpha brainwave activity. You might want to think of the way you look up at the screen in a movie theater, a comfortable upward angle.

3. Counting backward is relaxing. Counting forward is activating. 1–2–3 is like "get ready, get set, go!" 3–2–1 is pacifying. You are going nowhere except deeper within yourself.
4. Imagining yourself the way you want to be—while relaxed—creates the picture. Failures who relax and imagine themselves making mistakes and losing frequently create a mental picture that brings about failure. You will do the opposite. Your mental picture is one of success, and it will create what you desire: success.
5. Words repeated mentally—while relaxed—create the concepts they stand for. Pictures and words program the mind to make it so.

6–8. These last three steps are simply counting to 5 to end your session. Counting upward activates you, but it's still good to give yourself "orders" to become activated at the count of 5. Do this before you begin to count; do it again along the way; and do it again as you open your eyes.

Once you wake up tomorrow morning and prepare yourself for this exercise, it all works down to three steps:

1. Count backward from 100 to 1.
2. Imagine yourself successful.
3. Count yourself out 1 to 5, reminding yourself that you are wide awake, feeling fine, and in perfect health.

40 Days That Can Change Your Life for the Better

You know what to do tomorrow morning, but what about after that? Here is your training program:

- Count backward from 100 to 1 for 10 mornings.
- Count backward from 50 to 1 for 10 mornings.
- Count backward from 25 to 1 for 10 mornings.
- Count backward from 10 to 1 for 10 mornings.

After these 40 mornings of countdown relaxation practice, count backward only from 5 to 1 and begin to use your alpha level.

People have a tendency to be impatient, to want to move faster. Please resist this temptation and follow the instructions as written.

You must develop and acquire the ability to function consciously at alpha before the mental techniques will work properly for you. You must master the fundamentals first. We've been researching this field since 1944, longer than anyone else, and the techniques we have developed have helped millions of people worldwide to enjoy greater success and happiness, so please follow these simple instructions.

Appendix B

Save the Planet Project

José Silva made the script of the Silva Centering Exercise available under a "Creative Commons Attribution-Non-Commercial-No-Derivatives License" for non-commercial use, so feel free to copy it and use it to guide family, friends, and associates to level.

If you want to use it commercially, please contact us.

Here are his guidelines on how to read the Centering Exercise to someone.

HOW TO READ THE SILVA CENTERING EXERCISE

by José Silva

The Silva Centering Exercise helps people discover an inner dimension, a dimension that they can use to become healthier, luckier, and more successful in achieving their goals.

When a person learns to function from this inner dimension, the person automatically becomes more spiritual, more human, healthier, safer from accidents, and a more successful problem-solver.

In order for a person to use this inner dimension, the person needs to hear the Silva Centering Exercise a total of 10 hours, and to follow the simple directions in the mind exercise.

HOW TO PROCEED

The Silva Centering Exercise can be read for 10 hours in one day, or read once a day, or once a week.

Take time at the start and at the completion of reading the Silva Centering Exercise. Take a break between each reading of the exercise.

Keep a record of reading time until 10 hours has been accumulated by the listener.

You can read to one or to several persons at the same time.

HOW TO READ

When reading the Silva Centering Exercise, read in a relaxed, natural voice. Be close enough so that the listener can hear you comfortably. Read loud enough to be heard, and read as though you are reading to a seven-year-old child. Speak each word clearly and distinctly.

Have the listener assume a comfortable position. A sitting position is preferred, but the most important thing is to make sure the listener is comfortable. If uncomfortable, the listener will not relax as much and will not get as much benefit from the exercise.

Avoid distractions, such as loud outside noises. There should be enough light so you can read comfortably, but not extremely bright lights. If you wish, you can play the Alpha Sound (available at our website) gently in the background to help the person remain at the 10-cycles-per-second alpha brainwave level. Do not play music; the frequency of music is constantly changing, and we want the person's brain to beat at a steady 10 cycles per second.

If the person shows any signs of nervousness or appears to be uncomfortable, stop reading; tell them to relax and make themselves comfortable. When they are comfortable and ready, then continue.

Take your time when you read; there is no need to rush.

The complete script of the Centering Exercise is in Chapter 6.

More Books by These Authors

José Silva's Everyday ESP Master Course
Unlock Your Natural God-Given Intuition
Complete Step-by-Step Guide

Creative Coincidences
The Next Phase of Human Evolution
Influence the Coincidences in Your Life

José Silva's Choose Success Master Course
Unleash Your Genius Mind
Original Edition

Silva Mind Control Method Student Q&A

For more books and to follow these authors:
amazon.com/author/josesilva
amazon.com/author/edberndjr

More Resources

Visit our website for our extensive knowledge-based, authentic José Silva courses, Silva Instructors and classes, and more:
SilvaMethodUltraMind.com

www.ingramcontent.com/pod-product-compliance
Lightning Source LLC
Chambersburg PA
CBHW061731050726
47598CB00002B/441

* 9 7 8 1 7 2 2 5 0 7 6 8 8 *